TURIYATITA

The Higher Consciousness Beyond Turiya

Author: Ishan Kyan

Table of Contents

Table of Contents

Chapter One

Understanding four states of mind: waking, dreaming, deep sleep and samadhi

Many of the greatest yoga secrets in our lives and actions— the way we see, think, talk and breathe, over day, month, seasons and years— are concealed within our natural rhythms and acts. Perhaps the best of these mysteries is our continuous state of consciousness and its various levels. The consciousness is the very center of our lives, the constant inner light behind the changes of everyday life. We are essentially conscious beings who work through the tools of body and mind. Our present life is only one of many lives of the worlds of time and space in which we accumulate experiences. Understanding gives us the sense of self, feeling and understanding, which is the inner truth from which body and mind work. It's the core of our life.

Yet we are largely unaware of the meaning of our consciousness. We prepare our understanding of the external world so profoundly that we have forgotten its roots. Our difficult lives keep us from realizing who we really are, what (if any) survives death and what our ultimate goal is. Our outer image is stuck in us, which forgets our inner meaning of light. Our transient lives conceal our inner relationship with the Everlasting.

The effect of this diversion is that we are guided by external forces, not by internal awareness, into confusion, greed and sorrow. We live on our surface and rarely visit the peaceful depths of our being. In the dense material world, we seek outer satisfaction and we ignore the hidden joy within us. Our lives are a great mystery and creation of consciousness. This is our most important thing to learn. We should be motivated to research our own minds carefully, not just the outside world. We will explore the profound consequences of our day-to-day awareness changes by waking and sleep in search of self-knowledge. In the Indian spiritual tradition such an analysis has always been carried out, as shown on the preceding pages.

What Are the Four States of Consciousness?

Being aware is not just a metaphysical matter that is of no practical importance to us. It is the origin and the foundation of all our lives. The Indians understood that each day is a trip through the consciousness and spoke about four states: waking, dreaming, deep sleep, and a fourth state beyond that, generally referred to as non-rem sleep. We usually deal only with the waking state and its demands, but the sense, personality and interpretation of dream and deep sleep still remain.

Such two subtle states, from health to spirits, have a profound effect on us and should not be ignored.

The Waking State, Jagrat Avastha

We don't live in a single state of mind all day long. Through the waking, dreaming and sleep phases the definition of our consciousness radically changes. Through the five senses, the dreaming mind sees a vivid outside world. It seems safe and strong and can be objectively sensed by every one of us. Nevertheless, our waking experience varies from moments of clarity to intervals of confusion and darkness in relation to our feelings, emotion and focus. However, physical reality has by its very nature many changes, contradictions and is essentially temporary.

Dreaming, Svapna Avastha.

The dream state provides a vivid and colorful, quickly changing and subjective essence of the inner creative consciousness. Through dreams we build our own personal reality, with its own sense of time and space, but with very no lasting effect on our outer lives. We usually consider the world of dreaming impossible through comparison with the reality we give to the world of waking. Dreams and astral visions also have their own mystery and beauty. Most of us interpret the dream state as simply a condition in which we recollect our memories and subconscious patterns. Such patterns often have no significance, but sometimes we have essential dreams. We have sometimes inspired dreams that enrich our waking life. And maybe we've got dreams shattered, that we hate the state of vision. In the study of the dream state, only the desires and traumas of the waking state are reflected in psychoanalysis. Its work is confined to subconscious and unconscious consciousness states with little knowledge of the more complex levels of consciousness.

Sometimes fictional, surreal and meaningless to everyday life are dreams. However, there was much more that we learned in the West to dream and sleep. Indian spiritual awareness provides a sense of dreams that can help us live a better, more conscious life.

All in all, we still live in imagination, that means that we dream even when we are awake. Our awakening state is going too slowly and doesn't give us the kind of push that we're looking for. That makes it a fun pastime to explore the realms of imagination and vision. Today, technology brings us "virtual realities" and "increased reality," close to waking dream projections. People may soon like this abstract reality between waking and sleep, as it fulfills our dreams and desires, but

has more physical connections than the dream state. Those scientific miracles are now supernatural approaching.

Yoga tells us that a whole dream world is present and that we have a dream self with its own personality and life. This is our astral body that remains in our soul after our experience of death. Whilst we still remain in the astral state, many people only have a shallow awareness of it, though certain souls have a deep astral life all life long. Many of these internally conscious beings are writers, mystics, occultists and psychics.

We function with an objective world of collective karma during our waking time. In the dream state, we work with our personal ideas and imagination in a subjective world. That presents us with a dilemma. If we do not have our minds under control, the dream state can quickly degenerate into evil visions, clothing or links with a low astral world of chaos, aggression, longing, anger and hate. Our dream reality will remain confused without control of our emotions.

Deep Sleep, Sushupti Avastha

Deep sleep draws us into an unmanifested world, in which all is darkened and put again into its seed form. Deep sleep is easy to ignore but is the root and help for the waking and dreaming phases they can't function without. We are looking forward to the ultimate relaxation and recovery as we slumber. In deep sleep we all feel peace and relax, and achieve rebirth in our souls. In this state, we do not know ourselves, but keep only its existence or its race. We arouse the feeling that we slept well. Sleep is peaceful sleep, in which we are naturally happy in our intimate sheath, anandamaya kosha, which also gives us access to the sambadhis or savikalpas.

The essence of our human incarnation lies in deep sleep, in which we return, though unknowingly, to the divine source of our being.

In deep sleep we return to our inner self, where our strength and memories are refreshed and vitalized for another day. But the deep ignorance and forgetfulness of Maya, the world's dream, overtake our knowledge of night.

We barely know that we are in deep sleep as we forget to sleep properly, and tiredness and tiredness will overshadow everything else we do. If there is no proper deep sleep, the mind and the prana, along with the biological moods– starting with vata dosha, the central motivating physiological force– will get imbalanced, which causes our organic structure to slowly collapse. Deep sleep balances our pranas and motivates us in our deeper resilience, which in ayurvedic philosophy is known as ojas, without which our force is unstable and diminished. Our immunity and perseverance collapse without deep sleep which ultimately causes the collapse of our mind and body.

Deep sleep, as the muleavidia or the' heart ignorance' of our lives, is understood in a Vedantic thinking. This poses the key barrier to higher awareness. The greater truth of the universal consciousness inside us is a kind of mystery or unknown. Moreover, if we learn to analyze this, appreciate and step beyond it, then it is also a major potential path to freedom of conscience. Deep sleep is the natural state of our samadhi or our harmony. The accuracy is tamasic. Nevertheless, it represents the samadhi qualities of peace and happiness, which can refresh the mind. Samadhi cultivation is a way to move deep and deep sleep meditation.

Until we begin deeper sleep, we remain bound by fate, wish, birth and death. We will not get deeper and more consciousness. We must live in darkness and unreality in the face of our inability to look into the inner light of truth beyond the darkness of deep sleep. Deep sleep is a metaphysical limitation, and not just a biological phenomenon. It's our life's central mystery. We shall not realize our true and celestial truth until we learn to awaken from this primitive darkness.

The essence of our consciousness on this side in deep sleep is Non-being, Darkness and Death. As we cross deep sleep into an ever waking consciousness, the inner light, light and immortality emerge. By crossing deep sleep, passing over death is not feasible. This is the alchemical path of the soul, which includes a transformation of our own core consciousness and identity.

Super consciousness, Turiya Avastha

More secret and enigmatic than these three ordinary states, is the capacity for ever-growing consciousness that is not subject to the daily fluctuations— the transcendent "fourth" or turiya in the yogic thought. This is the goal of higher yoga practices that take us beyond time and death. Turiya holds the true secret of our life, but we need to find out with absolute determination in order to unravel it. It is the unifying state of consciousness that underlies the three other states and transcends them. This description is in the Mandukya Upanishad, verse 7: "An intangible, impalpable, indefectible, inconceivable, unknown, whose nature is that awareness of the self, which absorbs all variation, is calm and benevolent. Without a second, what is called the fourth state — that's the atman. It must be understood that." (Vedic Awareness, p. 723). The fourth or ever-waking state is the samadhi's yogic consciousness, or conscience of unity.

This was explained by Sri Swami Chidananda (1917-2008), who said: "These three ever-changing conditions of awakens dreams, deep sleep is possible because there is pure consciousness or awareness. Thus, the help and substratum of the ever-recurring and always-changing triple or Avastha-traya state (three states of consciousness: waking, dreaming and deep sleep) is turiya Avastha (the fourth state), which is the Purusha (the Supreme Being) eternal principle of life- consciousness. The unchanging, everlasting knowledge of nature or sat-chit helps the three states. "The consciousness of creation implies super consciousness" (from the book of Swami: The Spiritual Life Trust Culture, Theory, Psychology and Praxis of Yoga, 1984). So, we can see that Creation-Consciousness-Bliss (Satchidananda) is the supreme state of consciousness and reality from the viewpoint of Advaita Vedanta.

This is also confirmed in Adi Shankara's commentary on the Mandukya Upanishad in the Encyclopedia of Hinduism (India Heritage Research Foundation, 2010). "Turiya is equal to Brahman, the highest self. It is the transcendent, ungual, all present, all-knowing, eternal, unchanging, self-effulgent, silent, inexpressible, absolute and ontological truth.... Turiya is defined as being beyond the three bodies and the five sheaths.... It is, therefore, the non-dual state of consciousness, free from all phenomena."

Chapter Two
Turiya or the Fourth State

Turiya or fourth state is the condition the human soul has to rest in during Sat-Chit-Ananda Svarupa or Nirvikalpa Samadhi, the higher Brahma consciousness. Three states, Jagrat, Svapna and Sushupti, exist for the Jiva in the mire of Samsara. Turiya is the disease that goes beyond all three of these countries. Therefore, the fourth or Turiya. Turiya is Brahman or Atman.

Brahman is the embodying of knowledge and happiness or Sat-Chit-Ananda Vigraha. He doesn't have a start or an end. He's the center of everything. He's for everyone a shelter, help and the Lord.

There are many languages, but one is the language of the heart and pictures. Cows have a lot of colour, but milk is one color. Many become prophets, but the essential things are the same in their instruction. There are many schools of philosophy, but the goal is one. There are many views and worship practices, but one is the Brahman or Lord.

The Self, i.e. the Pipeelika Marga and the Vihanga Marga, are both routes through yoga. Like the ant slowly goes, the aspirant also moves slowly on the spiritual journey. To purify his hands, he practices Karma Yoga and then Upasana takes his mind steadily. Eventually he follows Jnana Yoga's path and eventually achieves life's purpose. This is Marga or the Ant-Way of Pipeelika. Just like the bird flies in the sky, so the first-class candidate practices Jnana Yoga concurrently and becomes acquainted with the self. That's the bird path or the Vihanga Marga.

You may equate man with an installation. It grows and thrives like a plant and dies at the end, but not entirely. The plant is also growing, thriving and eventually dying. The seed that grows a new plant is left behind. Man leaves behind the good and bad deeds of his life as he dies his karma. The physical body can die and rot, but his memories do not perish. To enjoy the fruits of these deeds, he must be born again. Every life can be the first because it is the result of previous deeds, not the last, because in the next life it must be expiated. Samsara would therefore be without beginning and end, or phenomenal life. But for a free wise man, there's no samsara who lives in his own Sat Chit Ananda Svarupa. There is not one of them. The Samskaras, which brings him into this world twice, are killed by man by acquiring knowledge of the Self and by being freed.

Have a thorough Upanishads analysis. No such inspiring and beneficial research can be found all over the world as Upanishads. Each mantra has powerful, original, sublime and emotional thoughts pregnant. They are the creations of the universal Rishis of India's highest awareness. They give the readers warmth, inner strength, harmony and courage. They instill faith in the hopeless, strength in the poor, harmony in the cheerful and serenity in the restless. The Vedanta system comes from the Upanishads that comprise the ancient wisdom of the ancient sages. A thorough examination of these majestic Upanishads demonstrates clearly how large the Rishis of Year had been in the Heart. The Western scientists are paying tribute to the Rishis and appreciating the beauty and originality of the Upanishads.

Argue not. Give up physical warfare, gymnastics and clubbing. When you get into arguments and disputes, you will not be anywhere. Have living faith or unshaking belief, the words of your Preceptor and the Shrutis, in the life of the sinful, all-pervading Brahmin or the Eternal. Learn the basic principles of Advaita Vedanta from your preceptor. The Advaita Vedantin accepts six Pramanas, but Shrutis is the last court of appeal. Srutis includes the inspired observations and insights of the wise. In the following, he also opens his Vedantic speeches. Srutis Bhagavati says, "Ekameva Advitiyam, Brahma, Sarvam Khalvidam, Brahma, etc.." Sruti Bhagavati says, most logic and reasoning are not necessary to understand and know the truth. The truth is quite clear. It can be done by simple meditation. Mind is only a finite resource. It is an autonomous and a regular professorship. It is not autonomous and self-luminous. You're going to be fooled. Intuition is unfailing or unfailing.

These well-qualified and well-equipped candidates will really profit from renouncing or Nivrittimarga. Many give up the world and in temporary zeal take Sannyasa. We do not proceed on the spiritual way, as without spiritual life there is no training and qualifications.

The one who sits by physically calming his mind, who does nothing, is the most active person in the world; whereas the other who runs here and there and always is really busy, does nothing significantly. You may think this is paradoxical. Very few can say that.

Husk is normal to rice and rust to copper, but through efforts it disappears! Evan so Ajnana which clings to the Jiva or individual soul can be caused by the uninterrupted Atmic inquiry to disappear. Kill Avidya. Kill Avidya. -you remain in your own self incomparably strong!

Don't confuse Tandri with Savikalpa Samadhi and Nirvikalpa's deep sleep. Turiya and Huma are ineffable glories. The magnificence can not be represented. If your body is warm, if your mind is clear if you are content, know that you are meditating. If your body is heavy, you know that you slept while meditating, if your mind is quiet.

Death comes from ignorance and lust. The deathless or eternal Atman is done with experience. By experience. Eternal life as well as death sleep in the body. Life is a spark or a blast of lightning. Time is but death's blowjob. Sleep at Atman. Sleep at Atman. You're going to achieve salvation. Go over time. Go over time. You are going to reach heaven.

Drop the Indriyas. Fall Indriyas. Think about it. Meditate. Live by yourself. Live by yourself. The whole being is taken to a kind of rapture or divine pleasure. You are going to feel the joy of Heaven. Great peace is going to encircle you. In the seas of paradise, you'll be lost. Each wish must melt all names and forms into nothingness. Just everywhere can you look at the Self. This glorious state can not be represented. You will see it yourself. You will. Just as a stupid man can not express the joy of eating the sugar-candy, so you can not communicate the satisfaction of Samadhi or the Supreme Self. This condition is finite in terms. This experience is not ideal for language. It's the ultimate silence term. It is an everlasting mind's absolute silence. Peace has passed all understanding. Turiya or the fourth state.

State of Consciousness in Turiya and Turiyatita

What do holons from the inside look like? What you feel right now, whatever happens.

It gets a bit more complicated from there, however. The disparity between systems and states is one of the important differences AQAL highlights. In the most general sense, "Systems" is simply just another word for any degree (in any quadrant). Every level of a line has a patterned structure or. The patterned wholeness or phases are the constructs examined in structuralism and developmentalism, when perceived from without in an objective way. There are therefore, where Loevinger is concerned, certain essential constructs (or levels) of the ego's developmental line: "conformist, cautious," "individualist," etc.

(Such structures or levels occur in sequential phases so we often compare "structures" and "stages," but theoretically they are distinct, so we won't equate them in this discussion. Inelegant as it may be, when we mean the sequence of the development of zone 2 structures in the psyche, we are thinking about structural level. The development stages are Loevinger, Kegan, Selman, Perry, Broughton, etc.)

In this section we want to look into and compare and contrast the states of consciousness with those of consciousness— sterile as it may initially look like, this relationship is perhaps the key to the understanding of the nature of spiritual experiences (and therefore of the role played by faith in the modem and the postmodern world). Let's start with this humble and dumb introduction.

We said Zone 1 in the UL (indoor view of a T) is just what I hear, think, and feel right now. I should explain my present and immediate perceptions and fears in clear first-hand terms, and I would do just that by several forts of phenomenology ("There is a sensation of heaviness, heat, discomfort, lightness, affection, concern, exaltation and momentary experiential flashing etc."). These are all anomalies in Zone I approaches, some of which study other types of inner experience known as exceptional states.

What I experience instantly, as a first person, includes what often are called "phenomenal states" in addition to basic "contents," or "immerging experiences" – such as a feeling, a mind, an instinct, an image, etc. I never experience specifically something like "a conscious machine," although I may be in the stage at which all my thoughts are currently unknown to me within this setting. Structures can not be discovered only by zone 2 techniques, and meditation or contemplation of any kind can not be used to discover them. On the contrary, States are, under different circumstances, directly available for information. I have states, not structures, I realize.

Most of us realize consciousness nations, and so are the great principles of wisdom. For example, Vedanta gives five key natural consciousness conditions: waking, dreaming, deep sleep, testimonials (turiya) and nondual (turiyatita).

Altered or non-normal states, like exogenous states (i.e. induced drug) and endogenous States (i.e. qualified states such as meditative states), also occur in addition to regular or ordinary states.

Increased conditions are often known as peak encounters, both normal and non-ordinary.

There is a mapping of countries like, human, exogenous and endogenous states and possibly, of the great traditions.

Some of the meditation maps are extraordinarily complex, but are focused on Zone-I methods and guidance (e.g. zazen, shamanic travel, central prayers, vipassana) and can be verified by those interested in training as phenomenological experiences.

It is an interesting question (and that will be revisited, as this is one of the main areas of integral post metaphysics) that phenomenological encounters ('see, what seems like limitless light and love') have real ontological parallels ('there is divine foundation of being'). The psychedelic mapping Of Stan Grof is also a zone I mapping for those interested (which's why no zone 2 phases are included in any of its mapping).

Many major cultures have developed a complex psychology that goes along with these systems, and even if the specifics don't hold us back, let me highlight some significant features. The points that I am about to sum up are challenging and hard to prove in themselves. But for the moment we are just going to assume them. I will use Vedanta and Vajrayana as an example. We will have to begin with a complicated terminology (although Neoplatonism would be just as well).

The meditative states are different versions of natural states according to every one of them. For example, meditation with type is a variation in the dream status (Savikalpa Samadhi, for example), and meditation without form is a variation in deep sleep without form (nirvika / pa samadhl). In addition, three primary natural states (waking, dreaming or sleeping) accompanied by specific energy or' body,' (free gross body, subtle body, and causal body are said to sustain the testimony / nondual states) (e.g. Nirmanakaya, Sambhogakaya, and dharmakaya, respectively).

Although the terms "dirty," "subtle," and "causal" literally mean only species or energies (in the UR), we also apply to the corresponding state of consciousness (in the UL). Therefore, 5 major, natural and/or meditative consciousness states can be referred to as: extreme, subtle, causal, testimonial and non-dual states of consciousness. I frequently refer to 3, 4 or 5 separate states of consciousness, as practices do themselves– all 5 of which are intended).

The inference is clearly that for those of you who stopped trying to understand what I said somewhere in the middle of that essay, all men and women have at least five major states of consciousness which can all be encountered explicitly according to the great traditions of wisdom.

Subtle dream states, as I can experience in a vivid dream or a lively visualization exercise or in certain forms of meditation of shape, as in a vivid "day dream," or in the exercises of visualization;

Ever-present non-dual consciousness, which is not so much a condition as ever-present, is a state of deep sleep and of the kinds of shapeless contemplation and perception of total openness or emptiness; witnessing states or "the witness"— which is a witness to all other states, such as a capacity for unbroken concentration in a waking state and a potential for a clear vision.

The Vedanta and the Vajrayana hold that all human beings have access to these states and their corresponding bodies or realms by virtue of the precious human body.' This means that all humans at almost every stage of growth, also in their babies, have access to these major states, simply because even the babies are waking, dreaming and sleeping.

That's a very, very, very important point, that we will come back to.

(As a sneak preview, since the main contours are always present, you can have a full experience of a higher state but not of a higher stage. For instance, work in the awareness-raising stage of Jane Loevinger continues to show that you literally can not have a peak experience in a higher structure, such as the autonomous, but you can have a peak have of a major, subtle, causal, observing, or nondual state of consciousness. Exactly how we're going to want to return to these two suits together.)

While they are naturally and instinctively accessible to all humans, some of them are extensively educated or studied, and then they hold some surprises.

Chapter Three

Turiyatita, the State Beyond the Fourth

The Scriptures speak of a fifth condition ("after the fourth one") called the turiyatita. This is the deeper superconscious condition for some; it is beyond all levels of consciousness for others. The first describes it as being present in a witness state or as being purely conscious. For the latter, when we are fully formed in turiya, which has not been associated with the mind, we become turiatitis and finally have the greatest lack of experience with Nirvikalpa samadhi, samadhi without fluctuations, the highest form of self-realization. "There are five stages: Jagrat (waking); Svapna (dreaming), Sushupti (dreamless sleep), Turiya (the fourth) and Turiatit (beyond the fourth);" says the Mandala Brahmana Upanishad (2, 4-5). "These three stages of waking, of dreaming and of deep sleep are encountered by the Yogin, known as Vishwa, Taijasa and Prague, which are successive walks in these three states, not the Self." The Brahman is one who has performed Brahman, which is all-pervading beyond Turiya. Its goal, namely to emphasize this— that the Self is what is different from them and is their witness— is to call it the fourth (turiya). When we learn this, the three experts vanish and the belief that the Self is the fourth witness always disappears. This is why the Self is defined as beyond the Spiritual Instruction No. 8 "(turiyatita).

The scriptures speak also of the fifth state, Turiyatita. This is the highest superconscious state to some; it is beyond any consciousness for others. The first describes it as remaining in a witness ' state or purity of consciousness. For the latter, when we are formed in Turiya, and are no longer associated with the mind, we enter the state of Turiyatita and ultimately have the highest form of self-realization as a major lack of experience in Nirvikalpa samadhi, Samadhi without variation. "The five states (Avastha) are Jagrat (waking), Svapna (drawn), Sushupti (sleep without dreams), Turiya (fourth) and Turiyatita (beyond the fourth)," says the Mandala Brahmana Upanishad (2, 4- 5). The yogi is one who discovered that Brahman is all-round beyond Turiya." The experiencer of the three waking, dreaming and sleeping states, known as Vishwa, Taijasa and prajna who travel successively over these three states, Sri Ramana Maharishi describes. "The Self is not the experiencer. The purpose is to show that the self is what is other than it, and that it is the testimony of those countries, that it is called the fourth one (Turiya). When this is understood, the three experts will disappear and the belief that the Self is the fourth testimony will disappear. Therefore, beyond the Fourth Spiritual Instruction (Turiyatita)," no. 8 is identified as self.

In a state of blessedness, a devotee kneels his eyes to her Lord Siva who knits her in his hands' protected palm. In her centric and serene consciousness, she discerns his ideal reality internally and understands that in this world nothing is wrong. Her serenity bloomed in all four states, as she mastered yoga.

Sleep & Well-Being

Your biological time is not just a physical passage, but an inner passage in the consciousness mirrored. Your biological time is the period that passes through the day. It is established not simply by physiological forces, but ultimately connected to inner powers of immortality, from which we derive our ability to regenerate mind and body.

We wake up in the sunshine in the morning and sleep at night after the sun has set. Our biological clock represents the movement of the sun outwards. On the inside, the prana is established and the breath is measured in our biological clock. Everyday they breathe about 21,600 breaths, or one every 4 seconds, every 24 minutes or 1/60 of a day, with 360 breaths.

The mind travels with the wind and shares its variations and rhythm. The prana and the mind return to a retired state during sleep. Our organic clock is reset for another day in deep sleep.

Naturally, our modern behavior, which assessed our social events by mechanical clocks, has isolated us from the organic time of nature. We have lived in the night and usually stay up from dusk, counteracting our biological patterns, starting from the emergence of electricity. When we take our biological patterns, we are denied proper sleep, which will disrupt our physiological and psychological functions.

Our biological clock decrees that we live one day at a time with new experiences every day. Our body, spirit and ego are going through subtle changes day after day. Our life does not always pass in time, but is modulated or disrupted by day and night variations.

Every night during deep sleep our consciousness returns to a state unmanifest and returns in the morning, almost as if it were everyday death and rebirth. Our frequent retreat into hidden realms and our addiction of physical existence overwhelm us. This leads us to believe that our physical identity exists endlessly, which is not the case. During our daily walks, deeper forces of consciousness and infinity effect.

Often, one day at the same time, our spiritual practice gives us new opportunities to grow, to change and to recognize the increased awareness within and around us. Our spiritual life benefits from learning to accept every day's unique and changing power.

Mind & Prana

The four states change our minds and pranas dramatically. All mind and prana are engaged externally in the waking state. The mind is enmeshed in dual desire and repulsion currents like and dislike, enjoyment and pain, love and hate. The prana is inhaled in dual inhalation and exhalation waves, in sensation and in action and in the energy shift on the right and left corner.

The consciousness is removed in the dream state, and our prana turns inwards. Through his luminous visions and strength our inner mind emerges to drastically alter our perception in time and space. We also undergo a subtler non-physical prana, which transfers the mind's thoughts into a dream body. We work in the astral body, consisting of the pranamayas, the manomayas and the vijnanamayas koshas, when dreaming. Pranamaya dreams are primarily active in nature and instinctual. Visions of Manomaya are emotional and tactile. Vijnanamaya dreams lead to deeper understanding and cross into meditation like deep sleep.

The mind fuses to a state of latency in deep sleep. Prana upholds the body that upholds it from the heart. We undergo a natural deep pratyahara, a sensory retirement, in which all of our faculties return to their core capacity energy. (The Prashna Upanishad is a subject of discussion).

In the fourth condition, the prana and mind are combined into a deeper consciousness for those who are able to feel it through meditation. The spirit begins doing its own actions, which only operate as a unitary consciousness instrument and can no longer produce false operation. We must give up our affiliation with the body and remove the prana knot that binds with it to the fourth condition.

It is said that our consciousness resides in the eyes, in particular the right eye. It stays in the dream state in the ear. It resides in the heart in deep sleep— meaning the metaphysical heart deeper rather than the physical or emotional heart. It is based in the fourth state, but not consciously, as it is in deep sleep.

Healing

It is the root of all deeper healing to draw our prana or essential energy within us. In this respect, the deep sleep prana has the specific power to heal all other pranas and the mind. The brain is capable of removing negative habits and resources in deep sleep and resetting its equilibrium. For any psychological healing this is important.

However, the body's most profound healing is also the prana and the consciousness behind sleep. A yogi can access and guide this inner strength of a prana through the hands or eyes, guiding and healing his followers with it.

Sleep and the Home.

Most of us define our homes to sleep, to represent the value of sleep. The most private room in our room is our bedroom. We are all looking forward for a good night's rest, particularly after a busy day or after a long time off. It is a huge pain to have no room or place to sleep. The basis of our feelings of well-being is to build our home or place of rest. Sleeping in the same place gives us some inner satisfaction.

Nevertheless, it is not only a matter of a house, a space or a family. The sleep takes us back into our spiritual home, through which deep sleep renovates us with sacred energy and consciousness. The beneficial influence is felt by us all. If we have life challenges, we all want to go back to our quiet home and to the rest, to shut the world off, to relax and to let go — and to sleep well.

We are all glad to sleep, as we know that sleep takes us to a natural state of peace and stability that removes the world's cares. Bitch or king— both have fair night. Such deep sleep harmony will help us understand the harmony of our deeper consciousness. Nevertheless, it's not necessary to rest in our external home and let us learn to rest in the inner home.

Qualities of the States of Consciousness (Avastha)

The Great Cosmic Dream

Your lives are not a pure personal existence but our spirit, who has lived many lives in many different bodies and seen worlds. Your lives are a long time and a little sleep. Our physical life is based on the forgetfulness of our eternal origins and a transient external reality in which we lose our true spiritual identity and become the physical one only.

What is the length of our physical life? As long as a lifetime, most of us respond. The reality is that the status of sleep destroys our physical consciousness everyday. In sleeping conditions, we spend about 8 hours a day, or a third of our lives. It is much less the state of sleep than the waking state that we know. We do not take sleep seriously or treat sleep as true except as a waking state epiphenomenon. However, much is hidden in it, including the secret of the waking state.

The Fact of Impermanence

The vision is most typical of a momentary company, with no permanent result or stability in the outside world. You can't visit your waking dream sites. When a dream comes to an end, it is forgotten quickly. We may encounter huge success or great dreaming difficulties, but do not take them seriously when we wake up.

Although the waking state lasts longer than dreaming, there are similar time constraints. It's over, too, and we have to forget. The waking state is a type of lengthy collective vision. We have a waking world, which seems set in nature, which we call the material world. But if we take a close look, we can see that every second physical reality changes. Modern physics deconstructed physical reality and showed that in a vast and interconnected universe of space and light it was an illusion of subtle particles and energy fields. There are ongoing adjustments that show its illusionary existence behind the apparent stability of the material world.

The day's movement shows its transient nature, with morning and evening rapidly changing. One hour will go so quickly that we don't know it. The seasons change over the year is the main factor in the area of nature's transition and transformation. In the spring the outer rush of prana accompanies in the autumn its inner withdrawal. The most important thing is our own aging process through our biological timepiece that demonstrates that our physical body is a fluid movement, not a fixed fact. And our mind moves quicker, even in a matter of minutes or hours, than our body.

Our life's transience shows how dreamlike they are. Ultimately — however much we gain or lose can seem to last— they come to an end that will end like nothing, be it yesterday's food, the memories of our own childhood or the accomplishments of our adult life. The tragedy of the young people who die reflects the unpredictable transience of life. None of us can really be sure that this is not our last day.!

Most of us have encountered this reality of impermanence profoundly, for example in old families, and have realized that you have changed radically or are no longer. During the course of time, all of us loose our friends and family. Sometimes, as we grow older, the world loses interest in us. Even if great leaders of the world die, they too will be forgotten in a few weeks. Time's movement is constant and leaves nothing at all.

The sense of impermanence constitutes the cornerstone of great art and literature, particularly tragic events. We are all sad that we are actually going to die ourselves. But we do not see that our desire for eternal existence represents our soul's deeper and not time-bound truth. We must step beyond the illusion of time that comes about in the daily cycle of waking, dreaming and deep sleep, to find the immortal soul.

We forget our universal existence in the ignorance of deep sleep and slip into a minimal, outward consciously-looking consciousness. This is the amazement of the ego that allows us to take our physical body as our true nature and to forget the origins of consciousness within us. We stay in the shadow of the dark force of deep sleep by waking and dream.

The Illusion of the Senses.

It's a fact, or a phantasmagoria, that our physical senses placed together. Our visual sense gives us our main picture or perception of the universe. Sound provides interactions to us. More physical sensations like touch, taste and feeling.

Nevertheless, the senses do not give an insight into the true nature of things. Sensory pictures are symbolic and can easily activate our imagination, a dreamlike feature that projects fancy what our senses are seeing or what we want to do. For instance, the sight of a lovely woman has a different impact on the male sense than on the female. A starving man's smell of food is better than a man who has just eaten. Biological imperatives are activated by our senses and force us to act.

We spend a great deal of time evaluating our selected truth, whether it's what we buy, our relationships or are actually. Intelligence needs to develop to differentiate between how things appear and what they may be. Vedic philosophy teaches us that the entire world is a projection, a mirror image from a deeper consciousness.

Ishvara renders like Brahma. He sustains like Vishnu. Like Rudra, he gives everything back to himself. In this Ishvara directs the cycle of reincarnation like Trimurti when a person is incarnated, becomes manhood, then decreases into age and death, then he renaces and returns to the universe. The author maintains that every day is a conception, an evolution and a death, and we wake up in a new and different way every morning.

Our feeling is, in fact, as much a dream as it is a vision or cognition. The senses are as many visions and wish faculties as they are a way of determining objectively the meaning of any specific reality.

We all know about the famous story of five blind men who, because of their limited contact with it, each come to different conclusions on the existence of the elephant. The five senses remind us of the world that can darken or disturb us so much that clarity can come. We will try to understand who we really are behind the five senses and ephemeral physical organ as attentive perceivers.

Many people live in fantasy rather than strong awake consciousness during today's era of information technology. We invest our lives in virtual reality, social media pictures and digital bios to show us to others. Yes, it is easy to see the desire and imagination of our physical reality, but analyze our mental activity all day long.

Each Life Is a Day in the Lifetime of Our Soul

The regular movement from waking to dreaming and deep sleep represents our souls ' long transition from one life to another, or incarnation. Waking refers to the world of dense matter and nature, our stay in physical realm. In yogic theory, this involves the cosmos. Dream refers to our astral experience, the domain of subtle form, thought and energy. Sometimes in yogic theory this is called the Moon's atmospheric realm. Deep sleep involves our stay in the shapeless and causal realms of energy and light for the seed. In the teaching of Yogi (Prashna Upanishad), this relates to the heaven, the room or Sun.

Death and rebirth are much like sleep, vision and everyday reawakening. Death is but a night, with unshakable dreams and a new physical life finally awakens. We are born and died every day, so to speak. The self that wakes up in the morning varies somewhat from the self that was asleep the night before. Every night we leave something and every morning we take something new. The daily shift in behavior is most overlooked, but it is easy to see for those who are conscious. Try to think before you go to sleep in the night, and then consider it in the morning when you wake up. It is quite easy and not very common to have forgotten what it was.

Control of the daily movement from waking to sleep helps us master the larger journey of our souls through the physical, astral and causal worlds. We will conquer death and transcend all time and space if we can live one day in full consciousness. Day and night mysteries are deep.

Every Day as the Creation of the Entire Universe

Deep sleep is possible to identify with the center material of the cosmos, Mula Prakriti. We will penetrate to the center of life if we can stay conscious and observe it. Every day we can experience the evolution of the cosmos, from pure consciousness to materiality, via the cosmic Aum vibration.

The consciousness of Ishvara, maker, preserver and converter, with whom our soul is one, is behind the depth of sleep. That Ishvara makes and consumes everything is a daily experience. This Ishvara has been taught by the Yoga Sutras and the Adi Guru or original yoga teacher in the universal Aum vibration. This divine creative process is embodied in our individual soul.

Every moment in time, in fact, eternity is present. Every day and each night represent the overall time movement as Brahma's day and night. Day and night are its removal, or pralaya. Eternity is the infinite day of pure consciousness; whose dual shadows form our outer world of experience day and night. This will be our daily experience before we remove prejudice from our minds. Every space point is likewise the Infinite, which overflows with various brahmandas or cosmic eggs and exposes different world systems.

Chapter Four

TURIYATITA: Chidakasa in Cosmic Consciousness

In accordance with Natural Law, each human being is inherent in three attributes. These 3 attributes (Satva, Rajas, and Tamas) are purity, development, and inertia.

Each individual is encouraged to act when he is influenced by one of those prevailing qualities. This way every human being grows through an objective rule that guarantees that a person's actions under the rule of natural law have a just and proper reward. This leads to positive results and misdeeds to poor results for the worker concerned. If you are engaged in a spiritually intuitive quest, you will experience five separate states of mind.:

The first state is called the awake or conscious state.

The other state is perception or subconscious. We see everything around us, as we dream, constrained by the strength of our sensory organs, gravitating between the awakened and dreamed.

The third state is the state of' deep sleep.' If the mind goes through a state, we usually do not know anything about it. To pass over this state, the' deep sleep state' like' Gudakesa' has to have full control.

The fourth state is "Turiya," the "transcendental state" or the "serene and blessed state" supposedly learned by the mystic poets and saints. The' Turiya State' is governed by the natural law. Only someone who has thoroughly cleansed the mind should access this list.' Turiya is completely intuitive' and can only be learned in meditation or in confinement. See fourth position of the Tozan Five Ranks.

"Turiyatita" is the fifth state. In Turiyatita, when they entered a senseless space (Chidakasa) the great saints, including Hui-neng, the Sixth Patriarch of C'han and the Bhagavan Sri Ramana Maharshi, remain. Here, the Self or the one ceases to function, as the' mind vacuum' is a non- mentally vacuum, which never expresses itself. In this state we are not talking about a return to ourselves, as through grace of unmanifested spirituality it becomes one with the heart. Though the end results are the same, differences occur in the way these end results are accomplished.

TURIYATITA (Chidakasa): Zen master Tai-yung, wanting to pass by the retreat of another Zen master named Chih-huang, halted but during his visit politely asked, "I am told that you generally

enter into Samadhi. At the moment of such entrances, does your consciousness persist or are you still in a state of unconsciousness? If your awareness continues, all sentient beings are endowed with consciousness and can enter into Samadhi just like yourself. If, on the other hand, you are already in a state of unconsciousness, plants and rocks can incorporate into Samadhi." Huang replied, "When I enter into a Samadhi, I am not conscious of either condition." Yung said: "When you do not know any one condition, it is abiding by the eternal Samadhi, and it can not enter or come out of a Samadhi."

The combinations of Bhutakasa, Chitthakasa and Chidakasa were recorded as Vedanta. Bhutakasa is the body, and everything that the naked eye sees. Everything that is seen will vanish, that means that Bhutakasa is transient and ephemeral. Bhutakasa also takes the moon, the planets and the milky path miles from earth. Bhutakasa is made up of the rivers, seas, forests and mountains. All Bhutas (elements) and live creatures are made up. Chitthakasa is so vast that Bhutakasa is so swamped. The vastness of Chitthakasa can be very well imagined. A small part of Chitthakasa includes Bhutakasa consisting of the sun, stars, rivers, seas, etc. You can wonder how it can be. For example, whatever you see in your Chittha, for example, sun, stars, seas, mountains, etc. Often, you as a tiny entity compose the apparent universe. Bhutaka= s and Chitthakasa refer respectively to body and mind. For these two, there is a fundamental basis that the Vedanta calls Chidakasa. That's the same as the Atma. The three-Bhutakasa (body), Chitthakasa (mind), and Chidakasa (Atma), are a mixture of humans. The first refers to the one you believe to be, the second, the other, that you believe to be and the third, that you are.

Nature of man is everlasting and infinite. Such a human life is considered low and medium. The presence of Atma is denied as it can not be understood. The atma is symbolic of Chidakas. It's not built. It is unchanging and time and space transcends. This is mentioned in the Vedanta, namely Nirgunam, Niranj= anam, Sanathanan Niketanam, Nitya, Suddha, Buddha, Mukta, Nirmala Swarupinam (pure, final, attribute less, everlasting, sullied, enlightened, free and sacred embodiment). Bhutakasa correlates in Jagrat (waking state), Swapna Chitthakasa (dream state) and Sushupti Chidakasa (deep sleep). You have only happiness in Chidakasa.

Turiyatita

Still in mind– Outside Thought, Clear Consciousness with no Occlusions – Guru– The Freed Being– Moksha– Remain in Turiyatita consciousness.

Opid mind is called Turiyatita outside Turiya-there are four sates of being according to Hinduism.

Dream State, Sushupti, Deep Sleep, Turiya, Outside Deep Sleep. Beyond Deep Sleep. Above the fourth condition, Turiyatita the Avaduhta Upanishad talks.

Turiyatita is a stilled mind – Empty Mind –

The favorite text of Ramana, the Tripura Rahasya, would clearly outline the state of awareness and what is true MokSha or liberated beings Consciousness– Indeed, it's Turiyatita state– empty mind– still mind.

In Turiyatita state, ego identity consciousness is not Turiya state. In the Condition of Sushupti, the desire-power to speak afterwards, the self-consciousness that has encountered the Self through spoken words comprehended, still burns in the Waking Condition, and the Dream Condition experiences in a diverse way.

Bhagavan Sri Ramana Maharshi frequently quoted from Tripura Rahasya and thought that it is one of the greatest works to describe Advaita's traditional teachings. Still reading about it isn't enough– it can't be done simply by thought– or parroting it.

Why the Silence, why not Mind

There is a quote "Those who speak do not, and the ones who know don't speak." There are those who have come who have tried to express themselves... but they must still admit that there are not adequate terms. It is uncertain. Some people tried, but it is a lesson in futility... great works such as vivekchudamani and ashtavakra gita were tested.

Now the answer as to why it is impossible….

For the Word is felt... and the words and the emotions are technology... and technology is a duality.... Even those who are formless give just another shape. Mind and mind establish the Maya Kingdom of Form and Transient. That Which Is the Constant is beyond all division and duality and form.... So, when you say Maya it's coming into being....

How to meet now, so... This is why the Silence... external silence... why emotions and thought will cease.... Silence... Only then can you go beyond the mind... you can only enter the inaccessible...

in silence only... when mind and mind stop.... Then you go beyond what is... then you go beyond the temporary to the permanent.... -

The Mayan world ends in silence... in not thinking then true knowledge IS.... Reality is in pure consciousness.... The belief that you will cease to exist is unfounded.... for you will find that, while what is known as being personality ends... You must be willing to drop the world of passers-by you have so dear.... You're One in the pool of facts... You're what the transient world comes from.... You're the center of life, you're beyond creation... so if you wish personality and type, you'll...… That's Moksha... to realize, eventually, that you don't need anything to... That it was and is all only a game of mind in the ever-changing transient realms of desire and perception...

Realms... realms of desire and experience... The dream state of Maya...

Realization is not experiential.... Even though experience is the closest word of duality for reasons about being inside, experience has the beginning and end... and reality doesn't have the start or the finish. Self has never been born or ever been buried. You are unaffected by any form and Mayan experience.... The You of your

Self are untouched in the Mayan realm of dreams and minds in the night You of the Self...

Go to Quiet inside.... Only observe, drop the thinking... have no pre-conceptions... BE only!!!! Those who say don't speak– because you establish life in speaking... and those who speak don't know.... What is beyond growing language and duality theories. EOLBREAK

You break into ego form and are separated from the pure consciousness of Now Beyond Forms and Mayans.... You can't know if you're in rational thinking and mind functions in silence....

Live in silence beyond thinking and mind– you should live in silence until you enter it... but you will know that when desire comes again you will slip into the mind and Maya... but you will know it is only a game... therefore don't be afraid... Keep losing the delusions

Chapter Five
Atman and Turiya

According to the philosophy of the Hindu Advatic, spiritual evolution is an individual's conscious

effort to pass over the limited, visible, mind-body and intellect trio and reach an unlimited stage, the infinite spiritual stage, i.e. Atman. As per A. A. Atman is a living principle in man that transforms his inert matter (body, mind, and intellect) into a life being. Parthasarathy is the Symbolizing of the Hindu Gods and Rites in 1994. The Atman is always pure and unchangeable in Hindu philosophy.

Like Swami Sivananda expresses, I am the Athman, the embodiment of everlasting self-awareness, the changeless, which is pure conscious nature just as the character of the fire is heat, which is the working of the gross mind and the senses.

The Atman is One that shines with its own light, according to Sivananda. Atman is the one that shines various intellects just as the light reflects the light in the different water containers. The boundaries of waking, dreaming and deep sleep must be reached to the fourth stage called Turiya. You are shaped in Atman in Turiya. This is the original and real condition of man, his fundamental and everlasting being, the center of his personality. Through this condition, he tries to rid himself of his material needs and overcome them so that he can aspire to the real meaning of life. According to an example from Mandukya Upanishad, light does not require any other's services to enlighten this. Likewise, all other awareness will take the consciousness of its life, by order to know the Atman, since this is all actual object to be seen, but it is a state that can be achieved by complete self-understanding, complete consciousness and full knowledge. While Turiya is the stage that sets the Atman stage. Everything is understood and everything is seen.

The final step of complete dissolution is the death of the ego and the awakening of the spiritual consciousness. The "I," in reality, words, thoughts, body and desires, dies and takes over total consciousness. This awareness is a perception of the divinity of each one of us and the profound understanding that all beings are basically identical. We are all spiritually developing on different levels. And to achieve this level, the Turiya of the Hindu Advait and the 4th stage must be in the domain of the transformation. In this dimension, the Turiya and the fourth level can be interpreted as being identical. Realizing oneself would help one become the "mouthpiece of the Almighty," your "Ishta," and then one with Him eventually. "Atman and Parmatma are one," says Swami

Chinmayananda. Turiya is a state in which the "Subject" and the "Object" merge into the uniform mass of Pure Knowledge, the Knowledge Absolute. (1999: 92). Turiya is the fourth level, which is also clarified in terms of "vision" and "sleep." The spiritual sense of these words is confusion or not knowing the truth respectively. These words are used. Swami Chinmayananda adds further that the waking state (Jagrat) is not mentioned in particular because the waking state is part and parcel of the dream because both the waking and dream states are characterized by misunderstanding or misunderstanding of the truth. There is a misconceived understanding of reality whether one mistakes a cord to be a snake or a stick. Turiya is therefore beyond misunderstanding. Where no ambiguity, no misunderstandings exist Turiya is a state of total clarity. Again, sleep is used for failure to understand. The failure to understand the reality or not is the origin of a confusion in waking and dreaming states of the pluralistic, phenomenal universe. The non-apprehension is therefore both the origin and the confusion of the dream and the waking states.

The Turiya is also represented as an eternal state of "knowledge." Turiya is pure knowledge and knowledge as such is essential. "Reading" is Atman or Turiya. Turiya State is the state of in temporality.

In Mandukya Upanisad (2006), Karika, as Swami Chinmayananda replied; man, now lives in a state of sleep, under self-deception. Therefore, "When the trigger, ignorance of our own existence and the consequences of the pluralistic perception system both have been transcended, we shall perceive the truth in the fourth phase of our consciousness, Turiya." Complex knowledge is the happy moment of selfhood, a time of total enlightenment. It is an eternal, infinite, natural and total state of consciousness.

Swami Chinmayananda also states that man exists today as the all-pervading consciousness, not knowing the real being of himself. He says: This was his lot since its conception, the moment when the first unit of time came to be conceived. Therefore, life is beginning less (Anadi). We have been living in a state of sleep since conception until today, i.e. not knowing reality. When the ego fully awakens to the facts– the fact of its own nature, he awakens to the facts which is not dual, unborn, elegant and unspoken. The word "dreamless" implies that there is no misunderstanding of truth. The dream world of visions begins when we are awakened from sleep. Once we awaken to reality, every birth, restriction, ethics, and so on drops down, then ego once and for all dies, never again to rise up.

Chapter Six

Turiya and Turiyatita

Usually, Turiya is the undual, unconditional consciousness (see Gaudapada Mandukya Karika, for example). It is called pure consciousness, by Sri Ramana. It's Atman. This is Atman. Because it has "unconditional awareness," it is nirguNa brahman, also called the Para brahman.

Gaudapada describes that two aspects describe these three states of consciousness, namely the waking, dreaming, and sleepless (deep sleep).:

•"non-apprehension of reality"

•"mis-apprehension of reality".

' Turiya-Atman-Brahman,' means' truth.' Turiya is the unconditional consciously, the substratum for all three states, rather than a fourth state. Without a second she is the one, for realizing it and without knowing anything else.

Atman's failure to understand is the source of ignorance. Misunderstanding is the consequent consequence, which contributes to a pure consciousness of ourselves and the universe other than ourselves.

The lack of understanding of the seam is the reason for ignorance as to its true existence, for example in the cable and snake analogy often used in Vedanta. We make a mistake about a snake due to this failure to understand. The snake dies as soon as we understand that it is a real shell, since, apart from its substratum, there was no actual life for it. Similarly, because our true nature is mistaken, we erroneously identify with the consciousness of the body and see a separate entity universe. The sages tell us that when we understand our true nature, turiya, the duality between "I" and "other" (ego and world), and the non-dual brahman, is "experienced" as alone.

Sri Gaudapada gives us a useful way to see Turiya and the three States in his Mandukya Karika, and summarized what has been said above. Every one of them can be defined as follows:

turiya (Atman): non-apprehension of duality;

prajna (deep sleep): non-apprehension of Reality and of duality;

Taijasa (dream state): non-apprehension of and misapprehension of Reality;

vishva (waking state): non-apprehension of and misapprehension of Reality.

Turiyatita in the major Upanishads is not mentioned as far as I know. However, a few of the Upanishads minority include five states: vishva, Taijasa, prajna, turya and turiyatita. For instance.:

II.4. There are five Avastha-s: Jagrat (waking), Svapna (sleeping), Sushupti (sleeping without sleep), turya (fourth) and turyatita (beyond fourth) There are two....

II.5. The Yogin is one who has accomplished Brahman that is all over the world.

And

5. There is nothing more than Brahman of the five padas (i.e. the turyatita).

Sri Ramana Maharshi refers in a couple of instances even to turyatita, but he usually explains the conventional view. The way I understand that the connection to turyatita is not related to the traditional view of metaphysics, but to meditation. Most Samadhi forms (e.g. kevala nirvikalpa) do not fit into the 3 states very easily. It seems as if kevala nirvikalpa Samadhi is definitely not a "waking" or "dreaming," it also does not necessarily equate to' profound sleep.' It is not quite the same as overt Atman realization and therefore liberation, since the state is temporary.

The explanation, instead of four, for five states is that they are formed in the witness state to know that' I am' is not one of the other three. Maybe the term' turiya' is used here as a witness state for the fourth state. The spiritual aspirant, however, still has to realize himself as the non-dual Brahman– the fifth "ring." Hence the fourth latter stage (turiya) is called turyatita. So, when asked, Sri Ramana says, "Why is the self identified as both the fourth (turiya) state and the fourth (turyatita) state?" He replies:

"Turiya means the fourth one. The experts (jiva-s) who wander successively in these three states are not selves, but awake, dreaming and dreaming, known as vishva, Taijasa and pri-d~ na The aim is that the Selves is that which is different from it and which is the witness of these states, which is the fourth (turiya). It is the purpose of making this clear. Once we realize this, the three experiencers are absent and the illusion that the Self is the fourth witness is also gone. For this purpose, the Self is defined as above the fourth (turyatita)."

In the traditional way Sri Ramana refers to turiya, apart from one or two passages as mentioned above.:

What is turiya?

Just three states exist, awake, dreaming and sleeping. Turiya isn't a fourth; it's the three underlying. Nonetheless, people don't understand it readily. This is the fourth state and the only truth, it is therefore said. Actually, it is not alone, as it forms the substratum for all events; it is the one Truth; it is your very Self. The three states emerge on it as transient events and fall into it by themselves. So, they are incredible.

Both nirvana and turiya are ways of emptiness, but nirvana is the emptiness of space, and turiya is the emptiness of no space. The problem dealt with here is how their phenomenology varies.

You will recognize the difference between nirvana and turiya during sleep: when you sleep in nirvana and lose consciousness, the physical body sleeps in Turiya, but you remain conscious. There will be permanent awareness throughout those eight hours if a person goes to bed and lives in turiya for 8 hours. The difference between the vacuity of nirvana and the vacuity of turiya at night can therefore be seen easily.

But how do Nirvana and Turiya differ during the day? If you're in Nirvana and there's a sudden shift into Turie, the transition is striking: unexpectedly, the perception of space vacuum shifts to the awareness of vacuity and temporality. It means that consciousness can not move in space in practical terms any longer. As if you can't turn your head to the left or the right. your head is tight, immovable. It's then like the information center is completely quiet, while the environment looks in contrast like a tornado.

Chapter Seven
Turiya and turiyatita

References to turiya and turiyatita are usually metaphysical interpretations of what is and is not experienced by a person in such a state rather than phenomenological explanations. Therefore, the knowledge about these countries is quite limited.

Turiya is both non-dual and turiyatita. While turiya is often confused with the' source,' the two differ. Both states are formless, but causal processes are connected (there's a causal body). Turya forms are absolute (Turiya forms are not present). The absence of the cause is vacuum, whereas the vacuum of Turiya is void. The causal condition is highest, Turiya is not lowest.

As mentioned earlier in turiya, the consciousness is unbroken 24 hours a day. This doesn't always apply to jnana samadhi. When an individual is constantly in jnana samadhi, turiya gets totally dreamless.

Turiya and turiyatita are a condition of total clarity rather than an excited state like bhava samadhi. Turiya is an immaculate and eternal space, the unity of the Divine (Brahman). It is the root of consciousness.

You can be in turiya when you are awake, dreaming (but these will be "easy dreams") and sleeping without dreams. Staying fully aware during sleep, dreams (not even a couple of seconds) or twenty four hour, days or week or longer during the day, is not the same as sleep deprivation because, after two days without sleep or dreaming, people experience hallucinations. In Turiya, consciousness will live for days or more, but the physical body is fully rested and hallucinations will not occur later. Thinking processes are absent in Turiya as in jnana samadhi. It is possible to think in this state, but conscious effort is needed.

Krishnamurti, the "Source of All Energy," the Absolute's meaning [Mary Lutyens; Krishnamurti; years of fulfilment], is an illustration of the Turiya experience of mid- November, 1979.'

"K was to experience a further psychological encounter in India before the year ended. He gave a report of it to Mary at Ojai in February 21 1980, who did not visit India in the winter, referring in a third person to himself: on November 1, 1979 K left Brockwood in India [actually October 31]. He went straight to Rishi Valley after a few days in Madras. He had been waking with that strange meditation in the middle of the night for many years. He was trailing him for a long time. During his life, this was an ordinary thing. It's not a deliberate practice of thought, or a will to do anything unconsciously. This is uninvited and uninvited very simply. He listened closely because he remembered these meditations. And therefore, every meditation has a new and fresh quality. There is an unexpected and uninvited sensation of accumulating energy. It is so powerful sometimes to cause pain in the brain, and sometimes with fathomless intensity a sense of immense vacuum. He wakes up often with joy and happiness without calculation. These unique, naturally unpremeditated meditations grew intensely. They either stopped on the days of his trip or late night; or they had to get up and travel early. When the momentum came into Rishi in mid November 1979, he wakes up to find something entirely new and different one night in the peculiar quietness of that part of the world and in the silence untouched by the hoot of the owl. The movement had entered the energy source. This must in no cases be confused with the Brahman, who is the creation of the human mind out of fear and anxiety and the unyielding desire for total safety or even thinks of him as the deity or the highest concept. It's not all of that. Wish can't get it, words can't grasp it, and the thread of thought can't wind about it. One may ask with what faith do you say it is the energy source? You can only answer that with absolute humility.

Every night K waked up with this sense of the absolute all the time until the end of January 1980. It's not a state, a static, set, unmoving thing. This includes the whole world, human beings without count. After the whole body had recovered enough, when it returned to Ojai in February 1980, it was perceivable that nothing was left behind. It is the ultimate, the first, the last, the absolute. Just incredible vastness and exquisite elegance are heard."

Non-dual and B-levels

While the Non-Dual goes above every point, it requires a certain amount of spiritual development to be in a non-dual state. In "three stages of mysticism," this development is related to the B-line.

In "The Visuddhimagga: An Inner Space Map," Buddhaghosa said that this is the case:

"Nirodha [the non-dual state] is available to the nonturner or the arhat only, and only if all eight jhanas have been mastered too. Neither the stream enterer (srotapatti) nor a once back (sacridagamin) has released the requisite super concentration to form the ego-bound attachments for Nirodha. Even the slightest sense of desire is an obstacle to achieving this state of complete nonoccurrence.

It is possible to create a non-dual Hierarchy. The following are: Level 8B: Non-dual peak;

Level 9B: Non-dual plateau; Level 10B: Turiya;

Level 11B: Turiyatita;

Level 12B: Turiyatita vision.

For non-dual interactions, a-levels are not enough. An individual must grow to B levels 8 to 12. The reasoning is that non-dual does not necessarily mean that subtle energies can be seen at these levels as at the C-levels.

A person must grow to level 7b for non-dual peak experience, a person must develop to level 9B for a non-dual plateau experience and a Turiya (non-dual) permanence must be developed at level 10B for Turiyatita to level 11B. For Turiyatita the individual must grow to level 12B for a vision of Turiyatita.

Which explains why a simple, easy and essentially correct non-dual solution so often fails. Most find it the most straightforward or the best approach. This may be correct, but only if a stabilization has already taken place at a high level of development will a non-dual State be possible.

About the differences between turiya and turiyatita

Turiya is the Full harmony. Turiyatita is harmony with the Absolute and also is linked to all levels by the observer.

If the observer went beyond the trigger into turiya during sleep (while the body was asleep), the visual perception would be completely absent: no hallucinations, no visions, no subtle energy fields would be seen in this state.

For turiyatita vision this is quite special, for eight hours of constant awareness during sleep suggesting eight hours of visual perception. This kind of visual perception, however, is very different from normal vision. This is not an out- of- the-body experience. It is not a waking dream. There, inside and outside, there is no difference. It is also quite different from the' entoptic' (mainly two-dimensional, no-depth, and not-scannable phenomena created by the central nervous system, the brain, etc., that means they maintain their position with respect to the center of the field of vision if you move your eyes).

The fact that Turiya is "Atman" and Turiyatita is a perspective of "Brahman' is an important ontological distinction.

Examples of visual perception during turyatita

Perceptions are provided on all subtle (non-physical) levels at the macroscopic, microscopic and sub-microscopic level.

Sometimes spatial structures which has more than three dimensions can be perceived. Archetypical forces as well as Morphogenetic fields are now visible.

Force lines are seen as lines of light.

Visual perception is now located at a distance away from the physical body. Most times, there is a 360-degree field of vision.

Subatomic structures are seen, let's take for example, as if they are 40 cm high and at a distance of 3 meters.

All form structures on a subatomic level are now seen, not as solid forms but as lines of force.

It has been argued that the universe must be actively studied for its existence, according to the anthropically concepts of cosmology / theoretical physics. This deliberate awareness must work outside of space and time on all levels. This is Turiyatita understanding of experience.

The physical senses are mostly but not completely eliminated during turiyatita. You can hear and communicate with others while in this state.

In waking consciousness, it is possible to have Turiyatita vision, but the physical eye will not be working. Objects are seen in the subatomic level, yet you can not see the room in which you are, even with your eyes wide open. Normally, during night and sleep you will be in turiyatita because you tend to push turiyatita vision to the background by having to use your physical senses during the day.

1982 Yes Psych energy, v4 No. 4 "Sub-atomic particle extra-sensory perceptions: 1. Evidence and validity of current particle physics," (Science Publishers of Gordon & Breach Inc.,); 1983 ja Psych energy, v5 no. 1 "Subatomic particle sensory extra perception: 2. The unexplained explanation of fundamental particle structure" physical-mathematical analysis (Gordon & Breach Research Publishers, Inc.).

Phillips compared C.W. Theoretical physicist Stephen M. The observations made by Leadbeater in 1908 with quark knowledge available in 1970-80 suggested that, several years before its existence, Leadbeater had been describing subatomic particles (quarks) by theoretical physicist. If that is so, then there is evidence that there really is this kind of concept, just because nobody-not even a physicist-suspected these subatomic particles in 1908.

"Entangled minds"[Dean, Dean: "Entangled minds"] in Dean Radin's novel. There is the following incident, Paraview, New York 2006]: "Sir J.J. Francis Aston was employed by Thomson at the college of Cambridge (who discovered the electron). Aston read a book by the British Theosopher Annie Besant and Charles Leadbeater in 1908,' The Occult Chemistry.' Besant and Leadbeater outlined their vision of the internal structure of atoms in this book, which includes a new form of the element neon, which they called meta-neon. They reported that the atomic weight of meta- neon was 22.33. In 1912, during neon gas research, Aston noticed a material with this atomic weight. In a paper delivered at the annual meeting of the British Association for the Advancement of Science, he also called it meta-neon. The discovery of Aston was later named an' isotope' and became a crucial finding regarding nuclear structure...

There is evidence that turiyatita vision is used at the sub-atomic level, as stated here.

The Journal Physics World offers a more detailed summary of these tales, while Jeff Hughes ' article ' Occculism and the Atom: The Curious Isotope tale' is published in the September 2003 issue.

Dr Stephen M. Phillips (Cambridge University, UK and Ph. D. of the University of California, Los Angeles) has qualified as' Theoretical Physicist':

"Besant and Leadbeater later discovered in 1907 the neon-22 isotope by the psychic means five years just before the scientists found it…

… Due to the fact that most of their explanations of MPAs were published many years earlier only physical scientists believed that atoms had nuclei, Chadwick had discovered the neutron in 1932- twenty-four years after' Occulte Che' and had not been aware that they had scientific knowledge of protons, neutrons and masses because of the lack of any such facts. There is therefore no workable natural or alternative, unexplained explanation of why their 100 years old subatomic particles explanations would align with modern physics other than Besant and Leadbeater who actually use the ESP to represent aspects of the microscopic universe.

…The most persuasive form of ESP is undoubtedly demonstration of knowledge of some of the world's higher sensory aspects that several years later are verified in science, because this situation makes no space for doubt or logical explanation possible when the similarities between scientific facts and psychic experiences are so numerous and reliable as to offer chance to good fortune."

And:

"Siddhis or spiritual forces are mentioned in the Vedas and books on yoga which a yogi can attain by meditation, medicine, incantations or austerities. Eight of the Siddhis are identified by' The Yoga Sutras,' the first yoga exhibition written by Patanjali about 400 BC. In aphorism 3.26 of the Sutras he says that, by guiding the light of super physical faculty, a yogi can acquire knowledge of the young, the unseen or far off.:

The ability to acquire' an awareness of the unseen and the far-off' in parapsychological terminology (Puthoff & Targ. 1979) means the' remote view' of the whole universe. The desire to get' limited information' can also be seen as a distant view of the world of microscopy. It has the Sanskrit name Anima and is called' minuteness, the ability to become smaller than a sphere at will' in the Yoga script (Wood, 1965) [Stephen M. Phillips ' book;' Proof of a Siddhi Yogic, Anima, Remote observation of subatomic particles. 1996 Adyar]

Russell Targ an American physicist wrote:

"Annie Besant was associated with spiritual C in the 1890s. W. Leadbeater explains the arrangement of atoms in an inventive analysis. Leadbeater was the first person in the world to describe the distinctive nuclear structure of the three hydrogen isotopes in this early study at the English Theosophical Society. He wrote in his 1898 book Occult Chemistry that a certain hydrogen atom might have one, two, or three particles in its nucleus and still be hydrogen, with a clairvoyant sight. A scientist had still not discovered isotopes. Leadbeater was the first one to announce the survival of atoms of various atomic weights."

The yogic tradition defines "siddhis" — what are we call "body experiences," such as the capacity to go through walls and to walk in the air. The Siddhi, the beauty of the universe or the smallness of an atom, probably refers to the Turiyatita view.

Siddhis are divine, mystical, supernatural and otherwise psychic energies, abilities and achievements which are the result of spiritual progress by sadhana, such as meditation and yoga. Those who have completed one or several Siddhis are officially called siddhas. The achievement of Siddhis is typically independent, although many Siddhis emerge from the same conducive state of consciousness at the same time.

compare this to the Holy Spirit meets every new believer with a blessing, 1 Corinthians 12:4-12: St Paul explains. This gift could be intelligence, insight, faith, the potential for other people to heal, miracles, prophecies, spiritual discernment, language speaking or an understanding of an individual's words speaking in tongues.

The term "Shaivite" is currently being overused. For example, Iyer Brahmins are called Shaivites often, but they actually follow Smartha secta (which I'm discussing here and now), and adopt Shiva simply as their Ishta Devata. For example, they are Shaivites. Clear philosophic shaivism today is relatively rare (unlike a very recent

Vaishnavism). In my reply, I mentioned one specific Shaivite sect, the Basava Lingayat sect. Nonetheless, my question concerns a better-known shaivist religion, called Shaiva Siddhanta.

Just like the Sri Vaishnava sect is based on the Pancharatra Agamas, the Shaiva Siddhanta sect is based on the Shaiva Agamas and the 63 Nayanars poems. In any case, S.S. Suryanarayana Sastri states this about the Shaiva Agamas in this passage from his book "The Sivadvaita of Srikantha":

Yet a third view of the Agamas is that their object is to translate the Upanishads, that they establish the teaching of the latter and "that they bear the same connection to the Upanishads, as the New Testament of the Christian Holy Bible bears to its Old Testament." According this view, the Upanishads present the mission, and the Agamas its achievement ... Upanishadic knowledge moves up to the four states, of waking, dreaming, sleep and the fourth apart from these three: Agamic knowledge, however, extends to the turiyatita, which is beyond even the fourth.

The four states of consciousness are Mandukya Upanishad

You're referred to as Jagrat, or awakening, Svapna or dreaming, Susupti or deep sleep, Turiya or "supervision." Turiya is said to be a word of self-realization, at least from an Advaita perspective.

But the fifth word, "Turiyatita," intrigue me. I wonder, what scriptures are there about the condition of Turiyatita? Was Sastri right to identify it by Shaiva Agamas? If so, what is Agamas Shaiva??

Ramana Maharshi, despite being an Advaitin, was an active follower of the Shaiva Agamas

Why is one's Self described as both the fourth state (turiya) and beyond the fourth state (turiyatita)?

Turiya means the fourth one. Experiencers (jivas) who wander successively in these three states are not the Self, the three states of sweeping, deep dreaming and sleep known as vishva, Taijasa and prajna. The purpose of making this clear, that the Self is the difference and the testimony of the States, is to call it the fourth (turiya). When we know that the three experiencers are gone and the idea that the Self is the fourth witness is gone. For this reason, the Self is described as above the fourth (Turiyatita).

I believe the idea is that the soul has self-fulfillment in the state of Turiya, but there is no more soul that can even realize themselves in Turiyatita since they are no longer after Moksha; it is similar to Bhazkaras Bhedabheda philosophy as I speak here. However, Tirumular as all the Nayanars worked in the Shaiva Agamas community, so it is all the more evidence that the notion of Turiyatita is present in the Shaiva Agamas.

But where is Turiyatita mentioned in the Shaiva Agamas? And in any other scriptures, including Agamas Pancharatra or Puranas, is this mentioned? To date I've only found the following: the

Mandalabrahmana Upanishad, five Avas Pasha (states), viz.: jāgra Pasha (waking), the Svapna (dreaming), sushup Pasha, the āhurya (fourth), or turya Pesa (beyond the fourth). The Mandalabrahmana Upanishad is the only guide.

Chapter Eight
Turiya State

Since we are incarnated beings, we have three states of consciousness; Turiya is a state that can be understood by yogis alone. These three countries are proof of the dual world and Turiya is proof of the monistic universe. The soul was born from a monistic source and was born in a dualistic world in a physical form. Turiya restores the monism from which we emerged.

Macro brahman, Maya brahman, and Avidya brahman: Transcendent Brahman is Pure Consciousness without attribution, so it is Macro brahman (Nirguna Brahman). Macro brahman Isvara is Maya brahman, or Maya's Macro brahman. Micro brahmans or Avidya brahmans are human beings with a load of Avidya (ignorance). Such eponyms have been invented by me to conveniently describe Brahman's three stages. It's Para brahman, or Highest Brahman, Macro brahman. Siva and Sakti are ensconced in a sheath to the Maya, Apara brahman (Sabda brahman). Parang-Bindu (similar half of the seed, two halves or cotyledons wrapped in tight skin or sheath) is the condition of Apara brahman. Siva and

63

Sakti polarization occurs within the sheath; it is identical to the Y- and X-chromosome polarized in Meiosis with Y and X gametes resulting. Siva and Sakti have a polarization which turns towards Siva for a long time, Parasaktimaya, Sakti (Unmuki). When Ham and Sa (Hamsa Mantra) erupted with the Maya sheath, Sakti suffered the drawbacks of Bindu, Bija and Nada. The progenitors of the universe are Bindu and Nada. Bija is the Mantra's Sacred Silver.

Since becoming Izvara, Brahman has four states, and has only meditating, knowing the first three states of consciousness with the 4th state.

Visva is the awakening state which requires recognizing external events and experiential duality. Awareness is changing externally. This is the perceived self that includes actions, reactions and dualities. His sandbox is the natural universe. AUM's sound A matches the waking state of Vaisvanara which means "all men." The leading God is Aniruddha, Pradyumna's son and Lord Krishna's nephew, one of the four Purushottama emanations, Vyūhas. Nine Visna forms are listed in Garuda Purana: Sudarsana, Hari, Acyuta, Trivikrama, Vasudeva, Pradyumna, Samskarsana, Aniruddha, and Ananta

If an aspirant meditates on Brahman, he returns to earth as a person and has an objective experience in the world.

Taijasa is the state of dreams where we enjoy subtle things. We feel pain and happiness; consciousness travels inwardly; the mind is creative and the dreams come from waking experiences. The self is briefly released from the scientific world. The mind is constantly engaged and the senses are passive and deactivated. This state is balanced by the sound U of AUM. He is one of the four emanations of Purushottama, the presiding deity is Pradyumna, the son of Lord Krishna and Rukmini.

When the candidate is thinking about Brahman in the state of Taijasa, he enters the Soma Loka (the Sphere of the Moon) subjective universe after he dies. He returns to earth to stay with people after his visit.

The following changes are based on the view of dream sleep by Joseph Campbell. (Page 70, Light Myths.)

Both visions in vision sleep, like films in which you see yourself, others and other things, are mind creations. Although you are dual (subject) on the one hand and he, she and it (objects) on the other, they are all one because they are your creative mind. You've created a vision, a plot, and an illusion. Life is also a dream, an illusion and a myth. Heaven, and heaven, and heaven, good and bad, god and soul, I, and I, and She, I, and I are one. The acts in the dream are your acts; the act, the act, the one, the one, and the one, the one, that is, and she's you because there's no one else.

Deep sleep is Prajna. There is no understood or expressed urge. The third quarter of the self is prajna, full of joy earned and happiness. Consciousness is calm and the external or internal events are not aware of them. It's a temporary state of deep sleep. The ideas are incubated until they are born, and are incubated unconsciously. This state of union with Brahman provides the duration of a temporary relief. It is Prajna consciousness, for it has no heterogeneous empirical world experience and only knows one homogenous mass of bliss. It's not heaven, but it's sweet. All joy is the Higher Self; all happiness is Brahman. There is no empirical information, but its seed is present. AUM's sound M suits the situation. He was Balarama emerged from the embryo transfer from the womb of Devaki to the womb of Rohini under the guidance of Yoga Maya force of the Lord. Samkarshana is the main god, one of the four Purushottama emanations. It was necessary to transfer embryos, because Mother uncle Kamsa killed six Devaki's men before, and after he heard a voice from the sky, he said he would be killed by Devaki's eighth man (Kamsa). Samkarshana means the separation of anything and, in this case, it refers to the actual process of extracting and moving the embryo from one womb to another.

If an aspirant reflects upon Brahman in general (all three or AUM parts), he goes, after his death, to the Sun's sphere from where he goes to Satya Loka, and becomes one with the Absolute. He is uniformed with all of the other people who join the Complete (without distinction).

Turiya is the Transcendental Divine Conscience. The fused sequences of Visva, Taijasa, and Prajna fuse. Turiya is attributes secure. It is santam, sivam and advaitam, for instructional purposes (peace, goodness and nondual). He is the Self or he is. There's no objective consciousness, and there's no seed. Ramana Maharishi calls this "Wakeful Sleep." While awake, Turiya is present and working in the perfect. There is an irreversible union with Brahman in Turiya: there is unity with Brahman. The spiritual unity is permanent. Four progressive states of Turiya are, one deeper and one deeper than the previous. This state corresponds with the silence which follows the Sound AUM. The Supreme Vasudeva himself is the leading deity; he is Vaus and Deva, meaning an inhabiting god. (See below, compared to Level one)

If an aspirant focus on Brahman, he becomes a non-dual Brahman in all his four parts (Silence).

Turiya is described as follows by Ramalingso Swamigal from Madras (1823 -1874 C.E.):' I have it.

The goal of the different forms of yoga is to reach this undifferentiated domain of consciousness while awake. Within our Western language, we have no equivalent to this definition. It has no name within India; it is simply called the fourth condition and is the fourth syllable letter (AUM), the degree of silence. Because all our terms apply to waking thoughts and logic, to dream pictures and logic, and to ignorance. It is the absolute silence; we have no terms for this but it is what we are....

The Indian word for this form is Isvara, "Lord". Each deity can be taken as this lord. The vision you have in your mind as that image of God, whether it is Yahweh, Shiva, Vishnu, Diosa or Christ or the Trinity, or Buddha's highest image, is what will be felt. Everybody's going to be OK. And what he sees is that jiva, the spirit of your very creation, through many incarnations. The subject looks at its own item here. The romantic theory or the second cakra finds its meaning here: God is the true Beloved, the Beloved for which our soul is concerned. And anything else is just an insight into what God's truth would be.

It is evident from this that each of the four consciousnesses has its own emanation, Aniruddha, Pradyumna, Samkarshana, and Vasudeva, as well as four Emanations (Vyūhas) from the Lord. (Note: Prakrti (the Bhutas) is the fifth entity which, as the other three of them, is not an emanation of Vasudeva. This fifth being is a divine material substitute. (Aniruddha is Kama's son (Rukmini's son) and Rati's son and Krishna's grandson. The embodiment of loving God Pradyumna, Kama. Taraka, the enemy of the Devas. The Devas hired Kama to entice Siva and Parvati to put together a son who would be the defeater of Taraka. (The story goes this way). In meditation Kama, the god of love fired love arrows at Siva. Siva was annoyed by the break and from His third eye burned Kama with the fire. Rati, Kama's wife, begged Siva to make her wife incarnate Pradyumna again.

First, Samkarshana (Ananta) the manifestation of the Lord who chairs the ego and kills, at the time of dissolution is Samkarshana, the first and the most powerful presiding Lord over Citta (reason).

The third Vyūhas, which is president of knowledge, intellect, and understanding, and life, is Pradyumna, the son of Krishna. Aniruddha is the fourth Vyūhas to control the consciousness, senses and livelihoods of the universe of beings.

The primary Vyūhas are arranged in lineage from left to right with no order but centrality granted to Krishna (Vasudeva) or His brother, Samkarshana (Baladeva): Pradyumna-Samkarshana- Vasudeva-Aniruddha (Emanations or Manifestations of Krishna). The creator, Pradyumna; Aniruddha; Samkarshana; and the supervisor and controlling power, Vasudeva is the destructor.

The divine deities and free souls in Vaikuntham have foursome Vyūhas ready to worship. The perfected souls know the vibhava (omnipresent) ways of rebirth. The archa type (picture or idol) are consecrated images and icons for the faithful to worship in the temples. The type of the vibhava and the archa is the same, first for the spiritually perfected and second for the devotees.

An exception in Thirnaraiyur

In the ceremonial wedding stance marrying Vanchulavalli Thaayaar (Lakshmi), the Naachiyar Koil in Thirunaraiyur near Kumbakonam in Tamil Nadu shows the Moolavar Thirunaraiyur Namb (main deity of Vishnu). The myth is that Goddess Lakshmi, in the shadow of the Vanchula Tree, was born of Sage Madhava. The Bhagavan, who was wedded by the Goddess Lakshmi, appeared in the form of the

Pancha Vyua (Sankarshan-Pradyumna-Aniruddha-Purushotama-Vasudeva). It is seen in the Sanctum Garbha Graham.

Grandson-Son-Brother-Self is the following form. Aniruddha-Pradyumna-Samkarshana- Vasudeva is:

Saiva Siddhanta points to another State beyond Turiya, which has two stages, namely Turiyatita, the Un-mesham consciousness, eye opening (Isvara Tattva has been achieved) and Nîmesha consciousness, the eyelid closing (Sadasiva Tattva has been achieved). Un-mesham's eye opening; Nimesha's eyes closed. The awareness and consciousness of Sadasiva is deeper and purge than that of Isvara Tattve (Un-mesham), the yogi is equal to the Siva as Siva reveals to the Yogi his goodness.

It is an evolutionary retrograde cycle (in opposite to the evolutionary descent of awareness from Super-consciousness to mero sub-consciousness and instinct on the animal), which is the homecoming of Jiva to the plane of Sasarara where Yoga enters through Turijatitta, for further journey towards the Super-conscious or Pure Consciousness source; The Yogi rises from Vidya Tattva through Isvara, Sadasiva, Sakti to Siva Tattva, and makes the mind purer and purer by the purest at Siva Tattva..

Kaly's devotee Ramprasad says that he would prefer sugar (Brahman) rather than sugar himself, though he achieved Turiyatita by becoming one with Brahman. He liked to be separated from Kali to adorate her, as unity with her does not require adoration.

The distinguishing points of the Absolute and God are: Brahman and Isvara; Turiya and Prajna.

Level One: The Utter, Brahman, Turiya and Silence after AUM are linked horizontally. Everything is Brahman Unperishable. Everything is thinking, all bliss, no dream, no movement, no name, no form, all light and everything utter rest.

Level Two: Lord, Isvara, Prajna and AUM are in the Unmanifest category and are the real realm of beings and matter. He is the Thread-Soul who moves through all the universe's souls. These are inventions of the unmistakable Brahman. With pure wisdom or Prague, Brahman becomes ISVARA OR PERSONAL God. In being Isvara Brahman does not decrease or cease to be. Isvara's principle is the inner guidance (controller) of all souls, or unmanifest, behind the Mula-Prakrti. Comparing this with deep sleep.

Level Three: Isvara is Hiranyagarbha's immediate cause, that is the world's embryo. If this embryo (a state of internalization compared to the dream state, thoughts, and possibilities) projects itself into time and space, we will get Virāt. Ramanuja says that Isvara is Cit and Acit's inner controller (subtle and responsive being and universe).

Level Four: The manifested state is like a waking state when the cycle of the embryo matures and becomes permanent. That is Vaisvanara's counterpart. = Visva + Nara= Entire, universal, complete, all+ Men= all men.

The Avyakta, Hiranyagarbha and Virat are the same as Turiyatita, Turiya, Susupti, Svapna, Jagrat,

When we return to sleep, science continues to try to understand why we have dreams (REM dreaming) to dreaming NREM). NREM= Sleep without quick eye movements. The newborn stays in REM sleep for many hours. Dreaming and REM are two entities; dreamless REM can occur in frontal lobe injuries and perceptive brain injuries. Dolphins sleep during half-brain swimming and half brain swimming in REM mode. Two hours of REM sleep, humans spend dreaming. Default kills rats just a few weeks quicker than REM sleep deprivation. Drugs can affect sleeping conditions.

In REM sleep the precocious babies and untimely animals spend longer periods. More REM sleep appears to be necessary, younger the brain. It is reasonable to believe that during REM sleep the newborns build new neural pathways and new neurons; in the first year, the baby's brain grows three times. Sleep REM is sleep vision. Have newborns a dream while sleeping in REM? It's guessing everyone. During REM sleep mind is involved, and transmitter brain chemistry, pontine acetylcholine sets the stage, while noradrenaline and serotonin, the chemicals next in the cascade sequence, stimulate the front brain to make a dream run; a dream lets you drive your car in dream sleep, but doesn't get you out of bed to get to your car and drive it, since REM sleep is correlated with muscle paralysis.. REM is a cholinergic disorder and a cause for dreams, when dreaming are dopamines. Dream drama includes intact frontal and perceptive cortex (Occipito-time-parietal crossing) and a motor cortex dream paralysis. Frontal cortex is a place of dream, but the visual and auditory cortex interprets the images, colors, odours, texture and sounds. The images and impressions are not fed from the outside world, but are produced internally and therefore the frontal cortex does not exercise judgment. Mental health requires REM sleep and physical health requires NREM.

In the absence of information of what people are doing, those with somnambulism may do complex activities. Automatism takes control of the actions which it may not have recollection of. Wakefulness and natural inhibitions and volitions are absent. It is dissociative, volition less motor agitation (mind-body dichotomy), arising at stages three and four of deep sleep. The psychomotor and other symptoms suggest unconscious epilepsy. This is not where unconstitutional automatism is being debated.

The Cit, the Laws, Hiranyagarbha and Isvara join Brahman when retrograde involution takes place. AUM crosses any point and is inaccessible. A is the waking state, U is the dream state, while M is the deep sleep. The silence following AUM is the State of Turiya. As Isvara and Brahman are adored by AUM.

The object of devotion or worship can be widespread: nature, smaller gods, personal gods, holy place, saintly artifacts, Saguna Brahman and Nirguna Brahman. Devotion is of various types and therefore results vary. For all such entities, the Self is identical. In accordance with the object of worship, the result of this worship or devotion can vary from earthly goods to achievement in certain efforts, such as graduated liberation, Samadhi, Jivanmukti, or Moksah. The choice of worship hinges on the devotee's mental composition and ability; not everyone can become a Jnana Yogi. You may be content with karma yoga, bakhti yoga, and sarnāgati, or Prapatti. The person is the same in the serpent-worshipper and the yogi who practice jnāna yoga, but it is determined by the excellence of the mind at both ends and in between, and they both possess the potential for eventual moksa. The Yogi see God in the Higher Self without qualities and does not see the worship of idols, Symbols and pictures that are a repository of the holy vibrations obtained during consecration. Tantrics believe, in the image or idol of the divine power which comes to life subsequently, that the conscience of the devotee awakens Sakti; that is Prana Prathistha, dwelling in the image of creation.

Jung says, "A symbol is therefore a living gestalt or a form— the total sum of a highly complex set of facts that our intellect can not conceivably address and therefore can not be articulated in any other way than using the image."

It contradicts other people's views (who we respect) that images, icons and idols are not to reflect Christ.

Chapter Nine
The Upanishad

Upanishads are old Sanskrit teaching texts and Hindu ideas some of which share religious traditions such as Buddhism and Jainism. They are ancient Sanskrit books. These are the part of Hinduisms oldest texts, the Vedas, dedicating themselves to meditation, philosophy, and spiritual knowledge; in other parts of the Vedas, mantras, blessings, rituals, sacrifices and ceremonies are concerned. The Upanishads played an important role in creating philosophical ideas for the ancient times Amongst the most influential literature in the history of Indian religions and culture. The Upanishads alone are well known in all Vedic literature and their fundamental concepts lie at the philosophical heart of Hinduism.

The Upanishads are commonly known as Vedānta. The Vedanta is known as "the last lines, sections of the Veda" and as "the focus of the Veda". In all the Upanishads, the concepts of Brahman (ultimate reality) and Gentman (soul, I), and "know that you are the best man" are central to their theme. The mukhya Upanishads, together with the Bhagavad Gita and the Brahmasutra, are a base for several later Vedanta schools, including two main monistic schools of Hindus.

There are over 200 Upanishads, the first twelve of which are the oldest and most significant and are the most significant Upanishads. The mukhya Upanishads are mostly found in the final part of the brahmanas and Aranyakas and have been recollected by every generation and spoken orally for centuries. The early Upanishads all date back to the Common Era, five of them possibly from a pre-Buddhist time of the 6th century BCE, which lasted from 322 BCE to 185 BCE. Of the others, 95 Upanishads belong to the canon of Muktika from the last centuries of the 1st millennium BCE to about the 15th century CE. In the early Modern and modern time new Upanishads, after the 108th canon among Muktika, were still composed, although they often dealt with subjects unrelated to the Vedas.

The Upanishads were translated to a Western audience at the beginning of the 19th century. The Upanishads greatly impressed him and called it "the highest development of human wisdom." Arthur Schopenhauer the parallels between Upanishad and major western philosopher were explored by Indologists in the Modern Age.

The Sanskrit term Upanisad (from upa "by" and ni-ṣad "sit down") translates to "sitting down near", referring to the student sitting down near the teacher while receiving spiritual knowledge. Other dictionary meanings include "esoteric doctrine" and "secret doctrine". Monier-Williams' Sanskrit Dictionary notes – "According to native authorities, Upanishad means setting to rest ignorance by revealing the knowledge of the supreme spirit."

The terms "Katha" and "Brihadaranyaka," means "knowing the self" or "knowing Brahma," Adi Shankaracharya describes in his commentary on Brihadaranyaka and Ka furiii Upanishad that the word "means" The term is found in many Upanishad's scriptures, like the fourth verse of 13th volume in Chandogya Upanishad's first chapter. In those verses Max Müller and Paul Deussen interpreted the term Upanishad as' secret doctrine,' while it was translated by Patrick Olivelle as' hidden relations,' by Robert Hume.

Muktika canon: major and minor Upanishads

Over 200 Upanishads are known, of which one, the Muktika Upanishad, was built up in 1656 and includes a list of 108 Canonical Upanishads. These were further split into Upanishad, aligned with shakti, sannyas, shaivism (the god Shiva), yoga and sāmānya (general and sometimes referred to as Sāmānya-Vedanta), and shaivism (the god Vishnua). These are also divided into the Shaktish.

Some Upanishads are called "sectarian" because they pose their ideas by a particular god or goddess of a different Hindu tradition, like Vishnu, Shiva, Shakti or a combination of those, like the Upanishad of Skanda. Such traditions tried to connect their Vedic texts, thus affirming the Upanishad, Čruti, in their language. Much of these secular Upanishads, for instance the Rudrahridaya Upanishad and the Mahanarayana Upanishad, contend that all the Hindu gods and goddesses are the same, that they are an all-embracing feature and manifestation of Brahman.

Mukhya Upanishads

It is possible to split the Mukhya Upanishads into sections. Brihadaranyaka and Chandogya, the oldest, are among the early ages.

Early in the middle of the 1th century BCE, the Aitareya, Kau Fastidieni and Taittiriya Upanishads date from around the 4th to 1st centuries BCE, approximately corresponding with earliest Sanskrit epics. There is a chronology suggesting that after the 5th century BC Aitareya, Taittiriya,

Kausitaki, Mundaka, Prasna, Katha Upanishads had an influence on the Buddha; another suggestion challenges the assumption and dates it regardless of the date of birth of buddha. Following these major Upanishads, Kena, Mandukya and Isa Upanishads are generally placed, but these are other scholars. There is little knowledge of the writers except those mentioned in the texts, such as Yajnavalkayva and Uddalaka. Occasionally, a number of women are also present, such as Gargi and Maitreyi, Yajnavalkayva's aunt.

Each of the major Upanishads may be affiliated with one of the four Vedas (shakhas) exegesis colleges. Several Shakhas, of which only a few remain, are said to exist. The modern Upanishads often have little connection to the Vedic corpus and have not been mentioned or commented upon by any great Vedanta philosopher: their language varies from that of the classical Upanishads, being less descriptive and more formalized. As a result, they are not difficult for the average reader to understand.

New Upanishads

The Upanishads have not been classified as recent ones, but have been discovered and written beyond the Muktika anthology of 108 Upanishads. In 1908, for example, Friedrich Schraders, who attributed it to the first Upanishad prose, revealed four previously unknown Upanishads in newly found manuscripts called Bashkala, Chhagaleya, Arsheya and Saunaka. The text of three of them was incomplete and incomplete, probably poorly preserved or corrupted, namely the Chhagaleya, Arsheya and Saunaka.

Ancient Upanishads have long been respected for Hindu tradition and writers of different sectarian texts have sought, by calling their texts Upanishads, to benefit from this reputation. Such hundreds of "new Upanishads" cover various topics from biology to rejection of sectarian theory. It consisted of the early modern era (~1600 CE) from the last decades of the first millennium BC. Although more than two dozen minor Upanishads date back to the previous 3.00 CE, many of these new texts with the title "Upanishad" came into being during the first half of the 2nd millennium CE. For example, the main Shakta Upanishads specifically discuss doctrinal and interpretative differences between the two main Tantric sects of a major shakticism known as Shri Vidya upasana. The many lists available for the authentic Shakta Upani Godads differ, representing the sect of their compilers, to prevent them from providing proof that they "locate" in the tantric tradition. The content of tantric texts weakens even their status as a Upani lifestyle. Sectarian texts like these are not considered shruti and thus the authority of the modern Upanishads is not recognized as a scripture in Hinduism.

The four Vedas– Rigvida, Samaveda, Yajurveda (the two main versions or Yajurveda Samhitas– are Shukla Yajurveda, Krishna Yajurveda, and Atharvaveda) all are related to Upanishads. During the modern era, the ancient Upanishads that were rooted in texts in the Vedas were removed from the Vedic layers of Brahman and Aranyaka, compiled into distinct texts and collected in Upanishads anthology. The lists are related to one of the four Upanishads and are many of them, and in all of India these lists are inconsistent with the Upanishads and the manner in which the newer Upanishads are supposedly assigned to the old Vedas. The list collected in South India was made the most popular by the 19th century based on Muktika Upanishad, and was written in Telugu. The 52 Upanishads were most famous in northern India.

The list of Muktika Upanishads contains 108 Upanishads the first thirteen as Mukhiyas, twenty like Sāmānya Vedanta, ten like Sannyasa, fourteen like Vaishnava, twelve as Shaiva and eight as

Shakta. Two as Yoga. The following table shows 108 Upanishads recorded in the Muktika. The most important and outstanding mukhya Upanishads are.

A plurality of worldviews characterized the Upanishadic era. While some Upanishads are considered to be' monitory,' others are dualist, including the Katha Upanishad. In comparison to the non-dualistic Upanishads at the base of its Vedanta school, Maitri is one of the Upanishads who tend toward dualism that form the classical Samkhya and the Yoga School of Hinduism. We have a variety of ideas.

The Upanishads have inspired Indian thought as well as faith and life since their conception, says Sarvepalli Radhakrishnan. Only because they were discovered (Shruti) are respected by the Upanishads, but because they provide compelling philosophical ideas. The Upanishads are treaties of Brahmanism that is facts of the absolute hidden truth. "It is a strictly personal effort to reach the facts" their analysis of philosophy presumes. Word is a road to liberation in the Upanishads, Radhakrishnan says, and pursuit of knowledge by way of life is the philosophy.

The Upanishads includes metaphysical theory sections which were at the heart of Indian traditions. Chandogya Upanishad, for instance, contains one of Ahimsa's (non-violence) earliest known concepts of ethics. In the most ancient Upanisads and a large number of later Upanishads are also discussion of other ethical principles such as

Damah (temperance) and self-restraint, Satya (truthfulness), Dāna (charity). The Brhadaranyaka Upanishad, the oldest Upanishad is stated likewise in the Karma doctrine.

Development of thought

Though rituals are underlined by the hymns of the Vedas and liturgical manuals are used by the Brahmas for these Vedic rituals, the Upanishad Spirit fundamentally opposes rituals. The older Upanishads also incorporated more and more violent ritual assaults. Everyone who adores a divinity other than themselves, in the Upanishad Brihadaranyaka, is considered a domestic animal of the gods. Those who indulge themselves in acts of sacrifice are paroled by the Upanishad Chandogya in a procession of dogs singing Om! Let's just sleep. Let's recover. God! -Om! Drink it Let's.

Kaushitaki Upanishad states that "the ritual of introspection" must be replaced by "external rituals such as Agnihotram offered in the morning and evening, and that" not rituals but knowledge should be the solicitude. "Mundaka Upanishad explains how people have been called upon, given rewards, terrified and deceived in sacrifices, oblations and pieces of religion. Mundaka subsequently argues that it's dumb and weak, because it makes no difference to the present and post-life existence of man, because it's like blind men leading the blind, it's a hallmark of self-denial and empty intelligence, naive ignorance like children's, a pointless artificial activity. The argument of Maitri Upanishad that all sacrifices in Maitrayana-

Brahmane are performed in the hope of finally preparing a man for meditation and bringing him to the awareness of Brahman. So, let this man meditate on the Self after he has placed these flames, and become total and complete.

Maitri Upanishad

In the oldest Upanishads the opposition to the practice is not explicit. At times, the Upanishads expand the task of the Aranyaka with a ritual allegorical and philosophical significance. The Brihadaranyaka, for instance, interprets horse sacrifice practice or allegorical Ashvamedha. It states that by sacrificing a horse, the over-lordship of the world can be acquired. Then it is said that only through the renunciation of the universe conceived as a horse can spiritual autonomy be achieved.

Similarly, the Vedic gods like Agni, Aditya, Indra, Rudra, Visnu, Brahma and others are in the Upanishads equaled with the ultimate, eternal and infinite Braham-Atman, God is identical with the self and is proclaimed to be everywhere in every human being and in every living creature. Ekam Eva Vitiyam or "one and the other and without a second" in Upanishads is the one reality or Ekam Sat of the Vedas. In the Upanishad, Brahman-Atman and self-realization develop as the road to the moksha (free life and freedom).

The thinkers of Upanishadic texts can, according to Jayatilleke, be divided into two classes. One community, which included early Upanishads and some mid- to late Upanishads, was made up of metaphysicians who used rational arguments to empirical experience to formulate their philosophical assumptions and speculations. The second group consists of many Upanishads, who professed theories based on yoga and personal experience. Yoga theory & practice is "not completely absent in the Early Upanishads," adds Jayatilleke. In these Upanishadic theories theory evolved within contrast with Buddhism, as a soul (Atman) is assumed to be the Upanishadic inquiry, while a Buddhist believes that there is no soul, states Jayatilleke.

Brahman and Atman

In the Upanishads Brahman and Atman are two ideals of prime importance. The Brahman is the ultimate reality and the Atman is the spirit. Brahman is the material explanation for what happens, accurate, formal and final. It is the all-encompassing, sexless, eternal, eternal truth and happiness, but the root of all transformation. Brahman, "is the eternal, manifested and non-manifest root, substance, center and destiny of all creation, the shapeless infinite substratum, from which the universe formed." "The creative concept that is known all over the World is Brahman in Hinduism," Paul Deussen says.".

The word Atman means a person's inner self, the souls, the divine spirits and every living thing, including animals and trees. In all Upanishads, the main idea is the Tetman, and its thematic focus is "Know your life." These texts say that not the body, the mind, or the ego, but Atman– "soul," or "self"– is the inner core of every person. Atman is the spiritual essence of every person, its very essence. She's young, old. Athman is what you are at the lowest level of your life.

Atman is the main topic of the Upanishads, but two different themes are expressed. The two are rather divergent. Younger Upanishads state Brahman (the Highest Truth, Universal Concept, Being-Consciousness-Bliss) is the same as Atman, while former Brahman state Upanishads, Atman, but not the same. These somewhat conflicting ideas had been synthesized and merged by Brahmasutra from Badarayana (100 BCE). The Brahman sutras render Atman and Brahman both distinct and non-different, according to Nakamura, a view that was later called bhedabheda. Koller says that Brahman sutras claim that Atman and Brahman are different on some levels, particularly during ignorance, but that Atman and Brahman are identical and non-different on the deepest level and in the state of self-realization. This ancient debate has developed into several dual and non- dual Hindu theories.

Reality and Maya

According to Mahadevan, the Upanishads present two different types of the non-dual Brahman- Atman. The one wherein the non-dual Brahman-Atman is the universe's all-inclusive field, and the other where empirical, evolving truth appears (Maya).

The Upanishads describe the world and human experience as an interplay of Purusha (the universal, unchanging concepts of awareness) and Prak litti. The first is a tribune, the latter as a tribune, and Maya. The Upanishads describe Atman as "true knowledge" (Vidya) and Mayan knowledge as "not true knowledge" (Avidya and Nescience, lack of consciousness, lack of genuine knowledge).

"The term Maya was translated as' illusion' in the Upanishads, but then it does not include natural illusion," explains Hendrick Vroom. Myth' here doesn't mean that the world is not possible and is simply a human imagination construct. "To suggest, according to the Wendy Doniger" that the universe is an illusion (māyā) is not to say that the world is not possible; it is to say instead, that it is not what it seems, that it is something that is constantly being done. It means to be a reality, but a reality that we live through is deceptive in its true nature "Māyā does not just confuse people about what they claim to know; he limits their understanding more fundamentally.

Māyā is described in the Upanishads as the changing reality and he coexists with Brahman, the hidden true truth. Maya is an important idea for Upanishads, because the texts say it's Maya, which darken, confuses and distracts a person, in the human pursuit of happy and freeing self-knowledge.

Together with the Bhagavad Gita and the Brahmasutras, the Upanishads are one of the three principal origins of all Vedanta schools. The Upanishads have based their various interpretations on the variety of philosophical teachings. Vedanta schools strive to answer questions about atman and Brahman's relationship and about Brahman's relationship with the world. The Vedanta Schools are named after their friendship with Brahman:

There is no distinction, Advaita Vedanta says.

The jīvātman is a of Brahman, according to Vishishtadvaita, and is therefore related, but not identical.

All human souls (Jīvātmans) and matter, according to Dvaita, are immortal and separate beings.

Other schools in Vedanta include Dvaitadvaita of Nimbarka, Suddhadvaita of Vallabha and Bhedabheda of Chaitanya. The philosopher Adi Sankara wrote on 11 Upanishads of mukhya.

Advaita Vedanta

Advaita means non-duality literally and is a monistic theory of thought. This addresses Brahman and Atman's non-dual life. Advaita is the most influential sub-school of Hindu philosophy in the Vedanta School. In reflecting on the Upanishad comments, Gaudapada became the first person to reveal the fundamental principle of Advaita philosophy. Shankara (8th century CE), the Advaita ideas of Gaudapada, have been further developed. King declares that Mā Samukya Kārika, Gaudapadas principal work, is infused with Buddhism's philosophical terminology. King also notes that Shankara's writings are distinctly different from the

Brahmasutra, and many of Shankara's ideas contradict those of the Upanishads. Radhakrishnan, on the other hand, indicates that Shankara's view about Advaita was straightforward production by the Upanishads and Brahmasutra.

In the discussions of the philosophy of the Advaita Vedanta, Shankara referred to the early Upanishads to explain the major difference between Hinduism and Buddhism, arguing that the Hindu is Atman (Soul, Self).

The Upanishads contain four sentences, Mahāvākyas, which Shankara used to describe Atman's and Brahman's identity as scriptural truth:

"Prajñānam brahma" – Aitareya Upanishad - "Consciousness is Brahman" "Aham brahmāsmi" – Brihadaranyaka Upanishad - "I am Brahman"

"Tat tvam asi" – Chandogya Upanishad - "That Thou art"

"Ayamātmā brahma" – Mandukya Upanishad - "This Atman is Brahman"

While the Upanishads are supported by many different philosophical views, commentators have usually followed Adi Shankara in seeing idealist monism as the dominant force.

Vishishtadvaita

Vedanta is the second school to be established by Sri Ramanuja (CE 1017–1137) by Vishishtadvaita. Adi Shankara and Advaita School were disagreed by Sri Ramanuja. Visistadvaita is a philosophy of synthesis that bridges the monistic Vedanta Advaita and theistic Dvaita systems. Sri Ramanuja also quotes the Upanishads and says the base of the Upanishads is Vishishtadvaita.

The study of the Upanishad by Sri Ramanuja's Vishishtadvaita is a trained monism. Sri Ramanuja interprets Upanishadic literature in order to teach theory of body mind, "notes Jeaneane Fowler– professor of philosophy and religious studies, who has Brahman as his soul, his inner power, his immortality. The Upanishads are the same qualities as the Brahman according to the Vishishtadvaita School but are distinct in quantity.

The Upanishads are interpreted at Vishishtadvaita School in order to teach an Ishwar (vishnu), who is the seat of all good qualities, with all the empirically conceived universe, as the body of God that resides in all life. The school encourages a commitment to godliness and a daily recollecting of personal god's beauty and love. It brings you eventually to the essence of Brahman abstract. Through Sri Ramanuja's interpretation, "The Brahman in Upanishads is a living reality," Fowler says, "the atman of all life and beings.".

Dvaita

Madhvacharya (1199–1278 CE) founded the third school in Vedanta, the Dvaita school. The presentation of Upanishads was considered to be profoundly theistic philosophic. Compared to Adi Shankara's arguments for Advaita and Sri Ramanuja for Vishishtadvaita, Madhvacharya says his theistic Dvaita Vedanta is based on Upanishads.

Fowler states: "The Upanishads who speak of the soul like Brahman speak of resemblance and not individuality," according to the school of Dvaita. Madhvacharya interprets Upanishadic lessons of oneself as "entering Brahman," just like a drop in the ocean. It implies duality and dependency for the Dvaita school, in which Brahman and Atman are different realities. Brahman is a separate, autonomous, supreme Upanishad reality. According to Madhvacharya, atman only resembles the Brahman in a minimal, less dependent way.

Sri Ramanuja Vishishtadvaita and Shankara's Advaita school are both non-dual schools of Vedanta; both are premised on the belief that all souls will be able to hope and reach a state of happy liberation.

Chapter Ten
The Minor Upanishads.

The Vedas hold the leading position among the Hindu scriptures. The Upanishad, originating from the Aranyakas parts of the Aranyaka, was known as Vedanta, or the conclusion or final corona of the Vedas, because they were represented in the Araayas (Forest) after the learner had left the life of the earth. The word Vedas means, in accordance with its derivative C knowledge, "the end of all knowledge." Rightly, as his consciousness led an individual to Atma, the Upanishads were considered the meaning of life. The second part of the Vedas, in other words., Samhitas and Brahmana conferred upon man, if he were to comply with the requirements, only the mastery of the World which is undoubtedly inferior to Atma. It is these Upanishad that to the western philosopher Schopenhauer was the consolation of creation. "There are now, in all, 108 Upanishads, of which the principal or major 12 Upanishads referred to in 8'r1 8'ankaracharya and others were now translated to English language by Raja Rajenqra and Dr. Roer. This was later retranslated into the sacred book of the east by Max Muller together with another Upanishad named Maitruyu. Of the remaining 95 Upanishads, two or three have been published until now in English, but never as many as I am aware that is addressed here to the public. EOLBREAK

Many years ago, late Sundara Sastri, a good Sanskrit scholar, and I collaborated to make the Upanisad, which had not been tested before, into English garbs, and successfully published many of those Which in the monthly issues of The Theosophist. The Karmic agents wanted my late colleague to give up his clothes in the early age. Instead I decided to take up my earthly mission of promoting the cause of consumers for begging before the public the cause of God. I was not permitted to republish all of the above translators in a book form until the constant journey since then, £01 more than 18 years from place to place in every part of India. I am aware of the many shortcomings this book suffers and I have no hope that it will act as a groundbreaking piece that can lead real yoga's and scholars to enter the field and make a better translation possible.

There are several versions of the Upanishads to be located in Calcutta, Mumbai, Poona, South India and other locations. But we saw that the South Indian versions, which were practically the same in Telugu or Grantha characters, were in several cases fuller and much more intelligible and important. Hence, we embraced for our translation South Indian editions. The version of the 108 Upanishads which the late Tukaram Tatya of Mumbai had published in Devanagari characters approaches the South Indian edition. Since there are no £ 01 studies available in the South Indian edition of the Upanishads, I intend to have the recensions of this edition in Devanagari characters printed so that even those who have little Sanskrit knowledge can follow the original by using this translation.

Vedanta and Yoga Upanishads

The Upanishads which fall under Vedanta and Yoga are the more important, but the latter are the most secret in their existence, as they provide insights into the mysterious forces of nature and man, as well as into how they can be conquered. With regard to Veganta, its former teachers have rightly decreed that no one has the right to learn it until at least he has mastered Saghana Chatushtaya, or four means of salvation, to a slight degree. Through his philosophy, he should not only be persuaded that Atma is the only Truth and that all else is but the ephemeral things in the world, but he should in practice also have outgrown the desire for those worldly transitory things: he should also have built a reasonable influence over the body and mmd. Failure to meet these previous requirements leads people to multiple anomahs. By studying these Upanishads, the Orthodox and the clever without any practice have come into a bad difficult situation. Pilgrimages to sacred sites and to the Hindus rites, religious impurities at the time of birth and death, mantras and other things are brought to light in Upanishads such as Maifreya and others.' 1'0 Comments like these offer a gross shock to orthodox who are blind and rigid monitors and ceremonies. Upanishads are therefore not intended for people with this stamp. They are not meant for mere scholars who have no practical knowledge of them and have been immersed in worldly things. Some of us know how men with brains alone have transgressed the Mayan doctrine. Not just wise but unprincipled people actually try to justify all sorts of disagreements and corruption by saying that it is all Maya. The old Rshis knew full well that those who did not comply with its preceding terms would profane Veqanta. Only after the impulses and the self are conquered and the heart is pure, or the core knot is broken as Upanishadic writers put it, the atma is only fully realized in the heart: then is the atma realized in all the worlds too and then the world is known as Maya. But as long as the Atma is not realized by creation, the world is not realized as Maya, and "God in all" is in term.

In the Upanishad, a particular point worthy of attention is that not all the material on a topic is brought to the same level. A mass of materials and a number of Upanishads must be wade by if we can have a related view of a subject. Everything available information is given in a single place in modern times when a topic is taken up. Systemic way. Systemic way. But the Upanishads were not over 80.

Taking Prana as a concept that relates to life itself. One Upanishad provides one piece of information, another piece, and so on. And unfortunately, we can't have absolute and straightforward information about the subject until we read all together and resolve the apparently contradictory declaration. Perhaps because Rshis wanted to draw latent intellectual and spiritual capacities in the follower and not to make him a pure automaton, this method was adopted by the Rshis. At these moments, when knowledge is delivered in a good form, it is definitely easy to absorb, but it does not so much evocate the latent power of reasoning. Therefore, when the disciple went to the instructor to resolve a problem in ancient times, after hard thinking being unable to find it for itself, it was readily and permanently understood by the former training of the mind, and it also was reverently regarded as a blessing and a reward for the previously encountered difficulty. In addition to explaining the difficult points to the instructor, the teacher's job was to help him understand the things he wanted to learn. We can take the case of the soul as an example. Not only did the Guru clarify the complicated passages or points concerning the soul, but the disciple also left the body and the bodies as the soul. Although these gurus can not be made accessible today in the outside world, the only thing we have to do is ensure that basic treaties on Vedanta or Yoga matters are released in the public interest. I hope I will proceed in this direction in the near future.

As we study Vedanta and Yoga, we find other peculiarities that shed light on their grandeur. Every stressed those growth centers in the human body. The 12 main Upanishads and the Vedanta Upanishads written here deal only with the heart and the heart while many centers, including the heart, are dealt with by the yoga Upanishads. For simplification, all centers may be divided from navel to navel under the principal heading of the head, heart and part of the body.

Which, however? This seems to be the key to unlocking these secrets. The true man is the devil, and the soul will obey Him, all religions postulate. Through Christianity, God created the soul in His own image, and in order to reach Him, the soul must rise to the full stature of God. Hinduism says that Jivatma (the human soul) is an "Aman" or part of Paramatma, which is to unleash God's powers ultimately and compares it with God's sun ray, or a spark that comes from God's fire. Throughout both religions, there is a common belief that the soul is a manifestation of God with the pause of the forces of Christ. So first let's grasp God's qualities. He is reported to be all-pervading, all-knowing and powerful. Throughout Hinduism, these ideas are translated into Sat, Chit and Ananda. It is eternal life, infinite wisdom, and boundless power. The soul that interacts with the body assumes that it is working for the body's life: co-opted by the brain, imagines that it has only the brain-circumcised information, swept away by the enjoyment of the senses, whirles throughout the midst thereof as if it were a true blessing. But when she wakes up to the highest realm and looks up from the dream of the lower stuff of the earth, she uncovers her illusions to be of the same sort as the everlasting, all-knowing, and all-powerful God above him. And the human body in which its functions must make this discovery through the three mam centers of head, heart and navel by each soul m. It cuts through the heart and finds the heart knot when it learns the meaning of life; Through the brain, the pineal gland in the physical body, and its omniscience j by the nave, according to the Upanishad, is superior to the mystical strength known as kunundalina, which in itself gives it unlimited power-the force which is mastered only when a man arises. it is not only through the brain but through its highest position, i.e., Sahasrara. When Will is created to a large degree, obviously, 01' Omna, then it is said that, when it has been conquered, Kundalini leads to infinite powers and perfections, 01' Siddhis such as anima, etc., and that only by rising above the desires of the senses is Kuudalini conquers conquered? It is said by psychoanalysts that will contribute to will.

From the above it is clear that the Upanishads of Vedanta are only for those devotees of God who wish to grow the heart primarily and not of the brain and navel and that the Upanishads of Yoga are intended in their three aspects for all those who wish to have a full development of the soul. I may point out, here, that 8'ri 8'ankaracharya and other commentators commented on the 12 Upanishads only because of the supernatural existence of the other Upanishads who treat Kundalini, etc. not for all but only for the few selected that can initiate private activities. Had they also made comments on the minor Upanishads, they had to disclose those secrets that grant powers and therefore are not intended for everybody. The clues leading to the creation of these powers would be nothing but lethal to the societies. When it comes to dynamits, it can be traced to the perpetrator, as they are of a physical nature, but they can never be monitored by normal means if the higher powers are used by voluntary means. The ultimate truths which led to the realization of the higher powers are thus said to be transmitted by the guru to the disciple who has proved worthy after a number of births and trials in Upanishad called Yoga-Ku7J-dalini.

If he is an Adept, one who still has to edit and translate the Upanishad, particularly those who carry on Yoga, should be able to explain it. Sometimes the passages in Yoga Upanishads are very obscure, sometimes there is no name or verb, and we must fill the ellipses as well as possible.

Another point could be made about the Upanishads. It's said that every Upanishad is one of the Vedas. We can even assume that some of them are in current, even if we take the 12 Upanishads edited by Max Muller and others. Some, not Vedas. Why does that happen? To my opinion, this also confirms the Vishnu Purana's claim on the Vedas. At the end of each Dwapara Yuga, a Vega- Vyasa or compiler of the Vedas, as a Vishnu-e-small Avatare, embodies the Vedas. The Vedas were "all" but voluminous in the Yugas before Kali Yuga. Not until this Kali Yuga began, Krsbna- Dwaipayane Veda-Vyasa incarnated and removed the Vedas not appropriate for this yoga and its people, and broke up the remaining portions in four, with the aid of his disciples. So maybe we can not locate the Vedas that include some of the remaining Upanishads.

Chapter Eleven
Turiyatita Avaduhta Upanishad

Om! -Om! That's absolute (Brahman) and that's eternal (universe).
The infinite benefits from the endless. This then remains, as the
Absolute (Brahman), alone, holding the infinity of the Eternal
Universe. Oh, okay! -love be in me! In my environment, let there be
peace! Let the forces that work on me have calm!

Now, Adi Narayana (Lord Vishnu), the lord of all men (God
Brahma), approaching respectfully his wife, said, "What is the
Avaduhta way after the Turiya level, and what is its position? The
Lord Narayana replied to him. The wise think that whoever remains
in the Avadhuta track is rare and not many, if you are (the
Avadhuta), you are ever purified, he is in fact an incarnation of
dispassion, and indeed he is a visible form of wisdom. He is (really)
a great person, though his mind remains alone in me. I still live in
him, truly. As a hut-inhabitant, he entered a mendicant monk's stage
(Bahudaka) first; as a Hamsa ascetic, he reached a mendicant monk;
the Hamsa ascetic (then) became the highest level of ascetic
(Paramahamsa). (In this stage) he understands the whole world

99

through introspection (as not different from his Self), he refrains from any personal possessions in (a reservoir of) waters, (like) his emblematic staff, water bowl, wax tape and the ritualist duties put on him (in the previous stage, the secret points of his body); he is unclad (packed); Removing even the acceptance of discolored, dirty bark garments or (deer) peel; behaving afterwards as the subject to no mantras (i.e. conducting no rituals) and giving up rushing, oil wash, sandal paste on the forehead, etc... perpendicular to sandal powder, etc..

He is one terminating both religious and secular duties; free of religious merit or otherwise in all situations; giving up both knowledge and ignorance; overcoming (the power of) cold and fire, joy and suffering, honour and dishonour; having burnt up in advance, with the latent influence (vasana) of the body, etc., censure, praise, ambition, competition, ostentation, haughtiness, lust, hate, love, anger, covetousness, magical thinking, (gloating) joy, intolerance, envy, clinging to life, etc.; observing his body as a corpse, as it were; becoming self actualized effortlessly and unrestrainedly in gain or loss; sustaining his life (with food located in the mouth) like a cow; (satisfied) with (food) as it comes without fiercely longing for it; decreasing to ashes the host of reading and writing and scholarship; tasked with protecting his conduct (without vaunting his noble way of life); disowning the supremacy or inferiority (of any one); (firmly) established in non-duality (of the Self) which is the highest (principle) of all and which constitutes all within itself; treasuring the conviction,' There is sought else indistinguishable from me'; absorbing in the Self the fuel (of concept) other than the hidden known only by the gods; untouched by sorrow; unresponsive to (worldly) pleasure; free of urge for affection; Uncommitted everywhere to the momentous or the ignominious; with (the functioning of) all senses at complete stop; unmindful of the supremacy of his conduct, learning and moral relevance (dharma) acquired in the earlier stages of his life; giving up the conduct closely resembling caste and stage of life (Vanaprastha); dreamless, as night and day are the same to him; ever on the move all over; Left with the body alone left to him; his moisture-pot being the watering-place (only); ever reasonable (but) wandering alone as if he were a child, crazy person or ghost; always examining silence and deeply meditating on his Self, he has for his assistance the prop less (Brahman); This sage Turiyatita who enters the state of Avadhuta, ascetic and completely immersed into non duality (of Atman), gives up his body as he is merged with Om (the Pranava): ascetic is an Avadhuta; he fulfills the purpose of his existence. He forgot everything in keeping with the concentration of his Self (as well). The Upanishad, therefore, ends.

Oh, oh! The (Brahman) is endless, and the (universe) is endless. The eternal comes from the endless. It remains as the eternal (Brahman) alone, instead takes the infinitude of the infinite universe. Om! -Om! -love be in me! In my environment, let there be peace! Can the forces the work on me have calm!

Chapter Twelve
The Mandukya, Taittiriya and Chandogya Upanishads The Mandukya Upanishad

The Upanishad was named after the sage Mandukya who taught the most exalted, including waking, dreaming, profound sleep and the fourth, Turiya. The third and fourth states are marked by the enigmatic syllable Om. The Upanishad also takes great care that Turiya is not a country, because this would characterize it. We will start with that understanding.

The Upanishad seems to be the shortest verse of just 12. Besides its implicit philosophy, Gaudapada's commentary, entitled Karika, made it renowned. In the sixth century A.D. Gaudapada existed. And it's said to be a mentor, or Govindapada's teacher who has been Shankaracharya's most famous tutor. While Advaita's philosophy or non-dualism is really the message of Upanishads, Shankaran's school has an elaborate exposure and its systematization.

The seven limbs are also the "cosmic body" called "vaisvanara" rather than the human body. They are stated in verse V.18.2 of the Chandogya Upanishad, which we are discussing later on. "The heavens are his hands, the sole of his eyes, the air is also his breath, the fire of his heart, the water his belly, the earth his feet, and the body room" is a translation from that Chandogya verse. These are the seven limbs that are defined in the Mandukya Upanishad's opening verse and clearly include the manifest universe. The "mouths" of nineteen include the 5 sensory bodies, the 5 action bodies (to walk, to speak, to eject, to procreate and to handle), the five pranas, the mind, the intellect, the ego sense and thought (citta).

The Upanishad goes on. "The second is the dream state, cerebral internally, with its seven limbs and nineteen mouths as well. The verse informs us that in the inner dream world there are parallels to all we find on our outside. In this state one encounters the implicit sensations of the mind." What we are experiencing in the waking state, we do have dream conditions but clearly not the same environment.

"Deep sleep or sleep without dream (prajna) is the third stage. When the day's night's darkness and the external world seem to vanish, the unconscious curtain includes thought and understanding also in sleeplessness, and the mental's subtle thoughts seem to disappear. It's a mass of consciousness, it's laughing, its face is imagined. In this case, the person is said to be happy because there is no tension or conflict. Prajna rules over everything, understands everything and is the inner master. It is the source and purpose of everyone. The fourth, turiya, is neither cognitive, nor internal externally, but cognitive in both directions. It is not a mass of cognition, not of a cognitive one, not of a cognitive one, not of a visible, incapable of being spoken about, inconspicuous, without any distinctive characteristic, unthinkable, unnamable, the nature of the one-elf knowledge, the friendly one, the benevolent one, the non-dual one. This is the blackbird. This must be done.

Here we see a word that shows the disorder beyond deep sleep for the first time. The mechanisms of waking and dreaming are causal and effectual. Prajna or the state of deep sleep is the only trigger. The ultimate thing, turiya, is beyond reason. Gaudapada writes in his Karika, "Prajna or the state of deep sleep knows no other things. The real or the imagined doesn't know it. They know nothing. They know nothing. But Turiya, fourth, knew it all and always knew it." We are completely unconscious in prajna state. In Turiya, you are not aware and unaware. You are' super viewed.' There is one thing in common with Prajna and Turiya. Both do not have a fantastic world vision. Prajna is sleeping though because he is ignorant, while Turiya is free from ignorance.

Upanishad continues, "Atman symbolized with omkara, which has four parts, having defined these 3 States and turiya, the" power "underlying them all and transcending them as well. The akara, or Om's sound, is the wake power and is the source of apti, which means" to get "and adimatva, and which means" to get first.

"Everyone who knows this gets every urge and is the best of everything. Om's Ukara or U sound is the dream state, the root of the words utkarsa that mean' exaltation' and' intermediateness' is from ubhayatva. Who understands this, exemplifies and matches this concept in the strength of interpretation and consistency of knowledge? No one is born ignorant of Brahman is in his lineage,"

That needs to be explained. The waking state occupies the demonstrated world. There is no wish we can not satisfy if we truly understand the nature of this universe. Anyone absolutely understands this world is "the greatest of all." The first part of these verses is therefore plain. The second section is more profound. It includes dream state awareness. As stated in previous verse, in waking and dreaming states the realm of cause and effect is found. Modern psychoanalysis made a major attempt in an evaluation of dream state to comprehend behavior. The works of Carl Gustav Jung point to the "collective unconsciousness" where, whether we know this or not, archetypal images have a powerful influence over us. Therefore, in order to understand the waking state, the dream world must also be understood and that means "continuity of experience." Anyone who understands both of these is the same. The' lineage' in the verse is the series of students who learn from such a person. This legacy has a deeper philosophical dimension as none of these two consciousness systems can fully explain the nature of life.

The Upanishad states that' Prajna' is the state of deep sleep and is represented as makara or Om's m tone. This comes from the root mi, which means "to weigh" or "to combine." Anyone who understands all of this calculates, merges it into themselves. The fourth, turiya, is the silence of Om, the amatra which has no elements of which the universe is decided, fine, not double. So, Om is the atman syllable. Anyone who understands this knows Brahman.

Gaudapada's Karika is important to make the Mandukya Upanishad's initial systematic statement and at the same time to create the basis for advaita as instructed by Shankara. The Karika is well known for its example of "snake and chain." Gaudapada says that just as we recognize that dream image is simply our imagination, when we "wake" the consciousness of Brahman, we recognize that this world is simply our mental projection. "You see a cloth, at a dark place," writes Gaudapada, "but you don't know if you see a cloth. You're going to see a snake, a water pump, or something like that. These are all misunderstandings. There's just a cloth, you have the illusion that the fabric is a snake. "There's a great many other mirages because of this illusion. The snake does not live without the chain. The relationship between the world we see and Brahman is therefore exactly the same relationship between snake and rope. Likewise, the universe has no life apart from Brahman.' The distinction between all three countries and turiya is as is the disparity between the Waking and the Dream worlds.

The Taittiriya Upanishad

The Upanishad of Taittiriya is often referred to as the calling address because a list of ethical principles for life is given to the leaving students. It has also been well-known for its 5 layers, namely, food, breath, soul, soul, and happiness, or koshas of the human being. A "calculus of happiness" to the last Brahman is also delineated.

The Upanishad starts with a prayer for the teacher as well as for the taught person. One can see the tension on pronunciation from the second verse in those ancient times. "We are expounding pronunciation, letters, sounds, pitch, number, intensity or tension, joint and mixture. These are the pronunciation laws. It's a mix of this universe. The best variations are here. The earth is the first type. The latter form is heaven. The ether is the bond and the air are the connection."

Speech is the way the teacher communicates with the taught person. Therefore, voice, intonation and emphasis and variations of words are extremely important for a true meaning. Language is, in essence, the awareness of words combined, which in effect are sounds combinations. The combination description is therefore established for further analysis. The wise man explains how this idea is mirrored around us in the universe. The world starts because it is not distinct from the heavens but rather connected to the planet in space. As already pointed out, Brahman's teaching is the core of the Upanishad. Although it is beyond your imagination, you should extend your understanding of yourself and the entire world to grasp it.

"Now, knowledge is its relation, and the knowledge is the link," continues the sage, "the teacher is the prior form, the student is the latter form." In this verse the sage transmits to the student a celestial image in the light of teaching. It's a part of the universal cycle, not an isolated event. This dimension of meaning we must be conscious of.

Then there are verses that gave the Upanishad its subtitle as a' Call Address.' "Practice virtue," the sage instructs, "does not stop learning and teaching. Do not stop studying and teaching, practicing truth. Do not refrain from learning and teaching abstinence (tapas). Do not stop studying and teaching. Practice self-control. Practice tranquility, do not stop studying and teaching." Such verses are reverberative in the message Svadhyaya pravacane ca and imply "do not stop studying and teaching.". The famous Socrates statement: "Unexamined life is not worth living" provides a faint echo of this. We should always question ourselves, the world around us, and always keep from knowing. At the same time, we must remember that the transmission of information is part of a linking organic connection and that we must not avoid transmitting the legacy of knowing to future generations.

While explaining the importance of education, the sage advised his students not to neglect social duties: "Matr devo Bhava, pitr devo bhava, acarya devo Bhava, an antithi devo bhava." "Your mother should be a god to you, your father would be a god for you, your teacher would be a god to you and your guest a God to you." We always forget that the Mother is for our only protection, our only protector, our first teacher, for at least the formative years. After that, the dad comes, the coach, the visitor instead. Here is also the seed of a teaching which comes in the form of karma yoga in the Bhagavad Gita later whose key message is the science of practice.

The sage instructs his students very humbly, "There is good behavior. Don't copy our shortcomings. Just emulate in our practices what's great! Giving with faith, humility and compassion whatever you giving. If any concerns or suspicions about any matter arise, seek the advice of the learned and the wise and act accordingly after reflection. So, we should not be reckless about our behavior. This is the lesson. "If there is a question, we can consult the wise, (not the other, as Plato says), and then act accordingly. This is also said that the four' R's' are basic education. We need to teach reflection in while also teaching reading, writing and arithmetic. We may conclude from this passage that the ancients have been taught.

The sage now continues his comprehensive teaching on the quintuple nature of the universe. "All things originated from food (annam). We live by food alone, and food is considered as the curing herb. Those who adore Brahman for food receive food. The breath (prana) is all beings ' lives. Those who adore Brahman as life come to life. Mind (manas) is beyond air, and words can not touch Brahman. Knowledge (vijnana) is beyond mind. As Brahman, all gods adore Vijnana. Yet Brahman, the root of everything, is beyond Vijnana."

The five layers of personality are described here. The outside layer is the physical body, the second, the electric body (pranamaya kosha) the third layer is the intellectual body (manomaya kosha), the wisdom core, and then the blissful body (anandamaya kosha). the second layer is the electric body. The sage gives us the "calculus of bliss" in order to understand Brahman's bliss: "Let there be a beautiful and well-known youth, who is very strong and very swift, so that the whole universe may become his dominion. This is one unit of joy we must call. The peace of the gandharvas is hundred times the happiness of joy and happiness. The Upanishad continues its hierarchy sequence of ten stages, until he enters the bliss the Indra encounters, then Brhaspati and then Prajapati. The Upanishad continues its Hierarchical sequence of ten stages. Finally, the happiness of Brahman is 1010 times greater than that of the rich, beautiful youth, which has all the wealth of the world. But the joy of a Brahman knower, who is not hit by desire, is the same as that of Brahman."

When we think about ourselves, we tend to think about our own minds or at all. But we should focus on and "eat" another dimension of our personality. We know the wisdom "sheath" or sheet

that is very close to the "blissful sheath." The Upanishad therefore teaches that Brahman is not very far away, it is very near.

The Chandogya Upanishad

The name of Upanishad comes from the word chanda, which refers to a poetic meter. The essence of this Upanishad is the importance of language and singing in life, poetically articulated. "Speaking yields milk," she says, as she sets the course of our lives and is the basis of our food. After the "interior singing" in our air system has been pointed out, it underlines that we need to be mindful of it in all our chants and singing. Otherwise it humorously says,' If we do anything' heedlessly,' our head will fall down'.

This is one of the long Upanishads with a variety of tales to describe his lessons. Just as the Mandukya centered on Om, the Upanishad starts as a lute singing with an instruction to meditate on Om. The essence of all beings is earth,' continues,' water is the essence of the world, water is plants ' essence, the plants ' essence is a individual, speech is the meaning of one's being, the Rg Veda is the anthem of speech, the chanting is the essence of the anthem, udgith is the ultimate expression of chant. Om holds talk and breath together.

While the Upanishads teach us that Brahman goes beyond mind and language, they are also trying to tell us that it is similar in every air of our life, closer than nearby in the world around us and. A person's essence is language and how significant that is! What a person thinks, knows, feels in his / her speech is revealed. Breathing is an important factor in chat. The "heart singing" of Om puts speak and air together.

"The light (deva) and the dark (asura) interplay within this body. The gods believed the udgitha was sense of smell, but since we could detect good and evil things, it could not be. Then udgitha, the gods believed, was voice, but since we could say both good and bad words, it can not be. The gods thought udgitha was the sense of vision, but, as we can see good and evil, it couldn't be. Then the gods thought udgitha is sight, but because both good and bad can be heard, it cannot be. Then the gods considered udgitha was mind, but it can't be good or bad as we can imagine. Then udgitha as prana (life) was thought about and the gods realized that prana couldn't be penetrated by the dark.

In this series of verses, we see the student lead to see how everything, good and bad, is filled with duality, and then eventually, the prana is not, and thus we understand a Brahman side like that. Then the gods thought udditha as life (prana) and knew that darkness could not reach prana.

The Upanishad follows other guidelines as to how to meditate on this instruction. "Anyone like udgith should meditate on the sun. The sun knows no darkness just like the udgitha. You can meditate on the breathing like udgitha because it sings Om all the time. The song of the udgitha is like the vina (a stringed instrument). The song is about us too. The track's in the rain. The track is in the rivers. The track is in the seasons. The song is in the birds' and animal's sounds. As the branch holds all the leaves together, so is the whole of Om's speech. It's all Om truly".

The Upanishad's central argument is that "album" is an essential part of life and that the music has to be one. The poetic mood is a way towards a higher consciousness. This perception is knowledge-transcending. "Is one who writes poetry to describe anything in his book" My Reminiscence, "the Bengali poet and Nobel Prize-winner, Rabindranath Tagore? It is a feeling the seeks to find external form in a poem in the brain. There was an error. The only difficulty is that words have meaning. This is why the writers must turn around and change them in meters and in rhymes so that meaning is somewhat tested and can be conveyed.". "The main aim of teaching is not to explain, but to knock at the mental doors. There was a mistake. I can remember a lot of things that I didn't understand but were deeply moving. There was a mistake. Late in the afternoon, I was walking our house's terrace. There has been a mistake. I could see that the night had come through me; I had been washed off by its colors. There has been a mistake. I saw the world in its true nature now that the self was in the past... With Beauty and joy all over."

As the wise man continues, "The heart has five openings. Remembering Prasna Upanishad. The breath is prana, the breath is vyana, the breath is apana, the breath is saman and the breath is udana. You ought to think about it. There was a mistake. Yes, a person is anticipated. It is intended for the purpose."

Here are some excellent examples. A young boy who wanted to know went to a wise person to be taught. The wise man asked him, "What is your dad's name?" The kid answered, "I don't know my dad's name. When my mother served several people, I was born. Then the sage said," Nobody except a brahmin can talk such a damaging truth about oneself. I just know my name is Satyakama and my mother is Jabala. "I will teach you because you did not deviate from reality." An important

feature of this time is evident here. The true meaning of Brahmin is a genuine seeker of truth, not a caste difference.

A different way of instructing the sage is now coming. The wise man gives 400 lean cows to Satyakama, to be taken into the forest. Bring them back when they're a thousand. Satyakama then follows orders and one cow talks to him after a few years,' We are a thousand, so bring us back to your teacher. Satyakama was struck and said, "Translate for me, please." The cow replied, "East Brahman, and west Brahman, so I'm telling you about Brahman. Brahman is the north and the south is the same thing. So Satyakama went to the flames, and said," Please teach me, please." Then the Fire said, "Brahman is the world, so is the ocean and the sky. Then Satyakama came and said," Know me! "and the birds said," The sun and moon belong both to Brahman, and also to the lightning. The sun and moon, as it were, are part of the moon. When Satyakama took the cows back to the teacher, the wise man said, "Your face shines as a Brahman-knower. The teacher is Brahman, and so are hearing and sight and mind." Who's been teaching you? The wise man taught him then and nothing was left out. "Beings other than humans, but now I think you can show me.".

Vivekananda writes to us about the voices of cows, fire, birds, etcetera when he describes the significance of this story. "All of the voices inside us are the brilliant concept we see here as a virus. When we better understand these realities, we realize that the voice is in our own heart. There was a mistake. The second idea we have is to obey Brahman's wisdom. The fact was demonstrated by everything the students learned. There was a mistake. The world has been transformed, life has been transformed, the sun, the moon, the stars, the lightning. All those stories are based on the principle that invented symbolism can be good and helpful, but better symbols than anyone we can invent exist. The early thoughtlets spoke to this world. Birds spoke with them; animals were talking to them; the sun and the moon spoke with them and they learned things little by little and became in the center of nature. They did not learn the truth through cogitation, by the power of the reasoning, by selecting other people's brains and creating a great text, as in modern times, not even I did, through taking one of their writings and making a lengthy lecture, but by careful inquiry and exploration. the main method was by practicing and so it has always been. It is to practice first before knowledge.

The next question reminds us of the Mundaka Upanishad's opening question. The student asks, "Master, what does it all mean to learn that?" The sage answered: "This teaching is just as understood through understanding a clod of clay. It would bleed out of this mighty tree, but still live, if anyone struck the root. It would bleed, but still live, if someone were to strike in the middle. Being impregnated with the man it is strong, drinking and cheerful. The student presents it to me, and says, "Sir, it's here." "Break it." "It broke, Sir." "There's a break." "Sir," he says. "What do you see? Sir.' Split one of the grains.'" It's gone, sir." "What you see? What do you see? Sir? "Nothing, sir." "My dear, it great Nyagrodha tree has come forth out of that' nothing.' The atman, from which this entire universe has emerged is intangible, imperceptible."

Then a progressive meditation instruction is given. The sage Narada came to another sage, Sanatkumara, saying: "I studied all the fields of education, literature, science, music, philosophy, and sacred scripture. I've got no peace, however. The revered wise man Sanatkumara responds," What you studied is name only. I have learned from great teachers such as you, that only he who knows himself finds peace. "Think of Brahman's name."

What a great lesson! Note that all that Narada knows does not say is unsuccessful. By asking Brahman to meditate on that, He transforms and defiles it. Narada now asks, "Is anything more than name available?" The wise man responds,' Yeah, there's more talk than name. We know the many branches of learning by voice. Dream about Brahman's voice."

"Is something superior to speech?" This is a question of Narada. "The mind is higher than the words," answers the wise man. Both the word and speak can be held by the mind. "Is anything higher than mind? Meditate on mind, as Brahman." "Narada is asking." It's more will than mind, yes. If you want to, then you think, then you speak, then you utter the word. Thus, as Brahman, meditate on Will." "Is something higher? "Narada's asking." Yes, it's more than will to think. Although you know a lot, but you don't know how to think, you'll say he's nobody, no matter how he knows. Think about Brahman's thinking."

"Has something higher been there, sir?" Narada's concerned. "Indeed, contemplation exceeds thinking. As it were, the earth looks. The sky looks like it is. It looks like the mountains. By contemplation, anyone who has achieved greatness in this world has done so. The contemplation of Brahman requires a separate perception of a series of thoughts.

"Everything higher is there, sir?" Indeed, more knowledge and more understanding. Think about understanding and insight as Brahman. "The patterns arise from detached observations, and that is called the comprehension, that is to say, the perception of a pattern, the" law." "We are more important than knowledge and perspective. Hundred men of understanding will shake a man with both physical and mental energy. The world stands by power, indeed. The mountains stand by power, indeed. The world stands by power, indeed. Meditate on power as Brahman." "Power "here is to be regarded as a lasting effort.

"Nothing better is there, sir?" Food is more powerful than electricity. Neither physical strength or mental strength can be accomplished without nourishment. There is something better, sir? So, meditate on food than Brahman." "Food is greater than nourishment. Food is in Earth, in the soil, in the atmosphere, in the mountains, in the plants and in all life. All these kinds of waters are indeed. "Is there anything higher sir? Then, meditate on food as Brahman." "From food, heat is greater. It won't rain, and there is no water without the convection of heat. Think of Brahman on heat."

"Much higher is there, sir?" There's more room (akasa) than sun. Without room, there can be nothing. Sun, moon and stars lie in space. "That's something higher sir? Meditate on space as Brahman." "There is more space (akasa) than heat. Without space, there can be nothing. The sun, moon and stars lie in space." Is something higher, sir? Think about space as Brahman." "Yeah, more than knowledge, the desire is. Memory will not continue without intention. Memory knows while intoxicated by desire. "Is there anything higher than that, sir? Meditate as Brahman." Indeed, the prana of life is superior to wish. Prana moves breath. Prana moves breath. All this is Prana."

There are some items here that need explanation. We come here to very subtle, interesting thoughts. Through memory, the human memory is not intended, but the universal memory. The hypothesis is that creation takes place through cycles (kalpas) through Indian cosmology. The present universe is destroyed (pralaya), then another universe is formed (or, in reality, a projection). The theory says that the cycle continues cyclically. Where does the new universe live between creation and dissolution? It's in memory. Perhaps like Jung, we will call it the "collective unconscious," but the concept is the same. Where are the archetypes, until we appear in the realms of waking or dreams?

Vivekananda gives some further explanation of these points in his book on cosmology. We are honored. "All motion, all in the world, can be compared to waves that are rising and falling successively. Certain of these philosophers believe that for a time the entire universe settles down.

Others argue that this equilibrium is only true for structures ... What becomes of the world when it calms down? It exists in the form of origin, in finer forms only. There was a mistake. There's a lovely passage in the Rg Veda, the oldest human writing ever, and it's most poetical-' If there's neither something, nor nothing, if the darkness rolled over the sky, what lived? What? and it is given the answer,' Then there was a vibration less existence.' Then there was a prana but no motion; anidavatam means existed without vibration.' It'd escaped vibration. When the kalpa stops, the anti-vibrating atom begins vibrating, blowing when prana is given to akasa after blow. The atoms are condensed and various elements are formed as they are condensed. Such things are generally quite strangely interpreted: people don't go to philosophers or writers to explain them and don't have the brains to understand them. A stupid man reads three

Sanskrit letters and translates an entire book. If they go to the observers, they will find that it is not air or anything of that sort. They are translated as air, fire, etc. The akasa creates Vayu or Vibrations, works through repeated blows of prana. This Vayu vibrates, and increasing vibrations lead to friction causing hot tejas. Then the fire comes to a halt, apah. This liquid then gets solid. There was a mistake. Everything we know through movement, vibration, or thinking is a prana transition."

Chapter Thirteen
Sarvasar Upanishad

Understanding and being are the same thing. Being is the only way to understand. And there are two development dimensions: consciousness and life. More and more, you will learn and remain the same. BE more. Be more. BE more. The being has to grow; not awareness, not learned information-but it has to grow. There must be more knowledge, not knowledge. And only spiritual development is of consciousness. Anything but a burden that adds to your knowledge.

It's always dangerous to play with the realities, because they are going to destroy you. You are going to be born again. We have only been pregnant for years, life so life and not the conception. We are only pregnant, we are only a seed, because nobody is prepared to pay the price. And before you come to our searching joy, you have a deep misery to go through. This is a deep pain. You can't escape the pain of conception.

Why this prayer? The master's and the disciple's relationship are the closest bond possible, because not bodies but spirits are linked. It's

121

all bodily, even the mother and the son— it's just a physical connection. The lover's bond with the wife is still earthly. The only unearthly relation on earth is the relationship between a master and the follower. Then the master is lost when the disciple is lost.

With the ego, you're never free. All errors are born from the ego. Therefore, thinking that you are being rescued already means that you are still vulnerable. The more we learn, the less it is. The more we learn. The other shore is not just the unknown but the unknown. This is the mystery. It is this kind of intelligence that makes that mystical. This is mystery: you know and still don't know.

Like blood in the body, money is still circulating. Information can not be transferred like money; it is impossible to transfer the information. So, what should I do? What should the disciple do to the master? "Give us strength," the master prays. We should aspire together; we should aspire together, "but we shoot straight for TOGETHER. The master's family— a family member because they're not teachers.

Being a buddha is one thing, but being a master is an advantage. It's not as hard to communicate the truth to know. It is more difficult to communicate, because the other enters. You are alone in knowledge, but the other is in communication. And the other must be considered when you try to communicate. It's getting hard. So many people are illuminated, but there are not so many masters. What happened? What happened? The thing happened, it happened, but even the person is unable to understand the whole thing. The explosion happened. What happened What happened?

Seven days after his awakening, Buddha remained silent. Why does this happen? One of many explanations is this: he tried seven days to understand "What happened? What happened? Who did this occur to? What happened to, and who did it to? It's riverlike feeling. It persists and there is no end to it.

The correct enquiry starts with prayer; the enquiry is not real, otherwise. Doubt is only an illness without prayer. Doubt becomes only the form of inquiring and questioning with a prayerful mood and a priestly spirit. Ambiguity is perfect if there's trust inside. A positive sign is a real doubt. The lack of trust remains; doubt is only a tool. There can be no ambiguity. When ambiguity is the lack, then it's a never-ending retreat: you will start to doubt and doubt and doubt and there's no end to it. You continue to fall into greater indecisiveness, with doubt. Doubt must not be the goal to meet anywhere. Use it as a tool– it's beneficial, but keep your mind focused on faith. Doubt disappears.

There's a chance –you're gone. Doubt is therefore a self-destructive process; it's suicidal, for you are demanding and not open to receiving. You are not ready for the reply, but you inquire. You continue to ask and miss the answer to your question.

Prayer means welcome, celebrations– you are safe. You are responsive. Be available, ask, be free and ask. This UPANISHAD begins with the prayer, the enquiry and then the questioning of the God Force to help. Curiosity is not only about prayer challenging. It becomes a genuine quest with prayer.

The first thing about liberty is realizing that you're not safe. The first step, the fundamental thing, is to realize that you are in bondage. First comes the longing, then the urge is created; then you start to dream of liberty. But you have to realize that you're not free, you're a slave. The issue therefore begins: What is bondage? Intelligence is not slavery. The intelligence VIDYA isn't. Vidya means the strategies, the processes. "What is wealth?" What is intelligence, doesn't it mean? "What does the theory mean? Why do you do it? Why can you be free? Tell me the highest truth, the highest truth — for the highest truth is unborn. The fundamental truth, the fundamental truth, the greatest, the highest, is not to be born. The second, after you have been born, will die as soon as possible. False doors, pseudo processes with false keys are there. There are pseudo-Methods which means AVIDYA.

Dreaming is not only Dreaming; it's true, it's important. For explanations, you can't dream. There's a causality even of a dream. It's significant, it tells you something. Instead, it tells more about you and reveals more when you're big, because if you're waking you and others can deceive yourself and others, but you can't disappoint your dreams. Dreams are harder because we have not yet found a system for dreaming and dreaming with masks. The dreams are still naked, genuine; they show more truly the real face when you are awake than anyone you use.

And, this paradoxical thing that can happen: a dream becomes true, because you don't handle it, you don't– you're hilflose. You're true. A vision occurs; there is nothing you can do. You're not the doer, you can only be the watchman. You are completely helpless in a subtle manner. Due to this impotence, your dream gets real, genuine and reveals much about your mind. Vision is valuable to know and to ask. The UPANISHAD then asks, "What is this awake mind state? What is it that dreams? What's sleep that doesn't dream? And TURIYA is what it is?"

This term "turiya" only means "the fourth," and what is the fourth thing to be able to overcome all these three – alive, dreaming, deeply asleep? The fourth wasn't named; only the fourth, the turiya, was recognized because that is simply not a state of the mind, but of one's own existence.

These three are nations.... It is a land, a mode, a shape, a shape of your self, when you are awake. That's not what you're. It can adjust, it's an economy. You're going to dream in the dark. It is still a land of dreaming because it can adjust. You're going to be deep in sleep, sleepless– that's a disease too. Via "economy" something is meant to change and take. The fourth, the turiya, isn't the state. You're not able to change it, you're IT. Instead, the 4th starts and transcends them in all three nations. But the fourth thing is not really a state. So, what the four are??

The sociological perception that religion is born in a mind, is only nonsense, it's pure nonsense. You should understand that every god is born out of fear. No, no god is born out of fear— from love, from prayer, from a deep insight into the essence of being. Nevertheless, this viewpoint is supposed to be special. When others start to follow, they follow a dead ritual.

In a moment of openness and intense presentation, the sun can become sacred, when all of the five bodies have a profound opening and the inside is one with the outermost-even for a single moment.

Everything is only sacred in that exposition. Everything! ALL. Nothing remains in this exposition; everything in this exposure becomes just a benediction, a joy, a blessing. Matter disintegrates; all becomes alive.

Divisions break, there are no obstacles, cohesion is visible. From this peace, trust is born out of this love. Therefore, all sociological religion theories are ludicrous. Just the Logic is incomplete! But this is obvious, because the only thing in life is fear, the only feeling for someone who has not known love. Those are the basic experiences: you know either love or fear; you are expected to be focused in fear if your life is not oriented towards love. Therefore, the mind of men can only have two perceptions of the universe: one which focuses on fear and one which focuses on love. When oriented towards love, it becomes religion; if oriented towards fear, it becomes only a physical science. If you're afraid, you can start fighting.

Science is a challenge, a natural conquest, a victory, a battle– nature is the enemy. If life focuses on love– and this is a religious life– it's not a challenge. It is then a friendship, then an admiration; you aren't an enemy, and nature isn't an enemy. Then you have a deep friendship; then you are one. There's only one possible interpretation if you have not experienced deep love, love for all, then you can only perceive it through fear.

Chapter Fourteen

Conclusions

We lead common lives and don't know the latent divinity inside. We see them as our only reality, going through waking, dreaming and sleep states. Pujya Gurudevshri describes a fourth state of our consciousness while explaining the States and discusses how to manifest it for our spiritual enhancement.

The life of a human is described as the combination of three waking, dreaming and sleeping stages. You get up every morning and wake up, you get into the state of dreams when you go back at night and, when dreams stop, you get to the state of deep sleep. In this way, you spend your life, you have lived in those states since birth, and therefore you know these things.

Yoga is the state of Oneness where prana, mind, body, consciousness, inner and outer, inhalation and exhalation are all united. The illusions of the presence of the Earth, of mind, memories, boundaries, paths, gravity and all supporting mechanisms of delusion are crumbling down and creating a great fear which is overcome by a force of confidence in the words of truth.

The Scriptures speak of a fifth condition ("after the fourth one") called the turiyatita. This is the deeper superconscious condition for some; it is beyond all levels of consciousness for others. The first describes it as being present in a witness state or as being purely conscious. For the latter, when we are fully formed in turiya, which has not been associated with the mind, we become turiatitis and finally have the greatest lack of experience with Nirvikalpa samadhi, samadhi without fluctuations, the highest form of self-realization. "There are five stages: Jagrat (waking); Svapna (dreaming), Sushupti (dreamless sleep), Turiya (the fourth) and Turiatit (beyond the fourth);" says the Mandala Brahmana Upanishad. "These three stages of waking, of dreaming and of deep sleep are encountered by the Yogin, known as Vishwa, Taijasa and Prague, which are successive walks in these three states, not the Self." The Brahman is one who has performed Brahman, which is all- pervading beyond Turiya. Its goal, namely to emphasize this— that the Self is what is different from them and is their witness, is to call it the fourth (turiya).

All objective information limited to the protection and safety of every jivah and ego collapses and becomes disintegrated by the ever-growing energy and emerging wonders of the unknown. For the advent of Para Kundalini Sakti, the vision of the body and the universe is unlikely. The vision of the Great Dream (Maya) is shattered, collapsing, cracked, broken, gone.

Sakti brings Siva back to Turiyatita, a Great Rebirth, an awareness of the Highest Truth, an unbelievable divine level of union, awe– wonder– euphoria of seeing and being an absolute truth, a total absence of all tensions– full relaxation and absolute spontaneity, Sakti' Siva (who has momentarily forgotten His Essential Nature and dreamed of being an individual's soul), a pashu (bound Soul)....

Self-realization is extremely scary for the ego, because death for the ego and the well-known, secure universe exist in this intense strength. This is why almost everyone adheres to your, me, and the earth around perceptions of the truth. Ego wants to live; it wants to survive. The earth look is so compelling, of course, that it is real. We do not interpret this "plane" of infinite consciousness "as the individual soul whose body just died, we call this" universe, earth."

When a conscious awakening penetrates deeper into the inner dimensions of reality, into the cellular, atomic, sub-atomic, quantum realms of reality, a huge force is unleashed that can render the waking soul scared. This growing force is very frightening. Unprepared person (mind) is scared of release of this enormous energy and immediately tries to recover its customary state of normal perceptions (temporary safe). The extremely concentrated energy source is fear itself. If the waking soul has the courage, terror, fear and the power of anxiety, anxiety releases energy it releases.

Released energy gives rise to anxiety of further concentrated energy. One must have full confidence in the fact that God Absolute is the real Self– the indestructible unborn, eternally existing reality. You must totally give yourself to Divine Grace. You have to be willing to die, to lose sight, to lose sight, to lose control, to lose the power of the objective knowledge, to be completely destroyed by the Absolute Infinite Energy. Only then does the Force manifest itself as the Real Supreme Intellect. Everything has been washed away from fear, doubts, confusion, actions, tensions and tensions. And one is an entirely Free Self

www.ingramcontent.com/pod-product-compliance
Lightning Source LLC
Chambersburg PA
CBHW051025030426
42336CB00015B/2724